CW00547175

The Wild Genie

The Wild Genie

The Healing Power of Menstruation

A Handbook for Self Care

Alexandra Pope

SALLY MILNER PUBLISHING

First published in 2001 by
Sally Milner Publishing Pty Ltd
P O Box 2104
Bowral NSW 2576
Australia

© Alexandra Pope 2001

Design by Anna Warren, Warren Ventures P/L
Cover design by Eri Jinnaka
Author photograph by John Chesworth
Printed and bound in Australia

National Library of Australia
Cataloguing-in-Publication data:

Pope, Alexandra, 1953–.
    The wild genie : the healing power of menstruation

    Bibliography.
    Includes index.
    ISBN 1 86351 279 9.

    1. Menstruation. 2. Women – Health and hygiene. I. Title.
    (Series : Milner health series).

612.662

All rights reserved. No part of this publication may be reproduced; stored in a retrieval system or transmitted in any form or by any means, electronic, mechanical, photocopying, recording or otherwise, without prior written permission of the copyright holders.

Dedication

To my mother,
Elizabeth Pope

Alexandra Pope

Alexandra Pope is a psychotherapist and menstrual health educator, living in Sydney, Australia. She conducts workshops for women and guest lectures at naturopathic colleges. She is passionate about supporting the Feminine, nourishing soul life, celebrating women's strengths and protecting the environment.

Author's Note

The content of this book is intended for guidance only. I am not a medical practitioner — the information and suggestions I make are not meant to be prescriptive. Any attempt to treat a medical condition should always come under the direction of a qualified health practitioner, preferably one experienced in nutrition and other natural methods of healing. Neither the author nor the publisher accept responsibility for any consequences of a reader failing to take appropriate medical advice.

Although I own the Moonphase cloth pads business, I do not have commercial interest in any other organisation or product mentioned in this book.

Acknowledgements

The Wild Genie has been carried by many different forces both obvious and hidden. It has felt buoyed at all times. Help or information turning up at the right moment. I constantly had a sense of having to thank some unseen force. Call it the Wild Genie herself!

The stories of many women, often very painful yet so rich and telling, form the heart of this book. These women taught me that there is no neatly defined path to health and that each woman needs to become the expert on her own body. A big thank you to all the women who have come to my workshops, lectures, for therapy or simply passing conversation. I'm grateful for your willingness to share the depths of yourselves so freely. Some of these women's stories appear either under their own name or under a pseudonym. All the stories are true.

I would also like to thank Lynne Clune for offering the first home for my workshops and latterly Jane Svensson for their continued support of my work.

Heartfelt thanks to my dear friend Richard Penny, an intensely loyal ally in my suffering, and whose own emotional courage both supported and inspired me to go beyond surface realities to find meaning in my crazy symptoms. He also gave me useful critical feedback on my early writing on menstruation — not always very graciously received at the time!

Much gratitude goes to Mariana Moonsun, my therapist, who got me writing on menstruation in the first place, igniting my creative voice, the best medicine of all! And to Jacqueline French, lover of ideas and passionate discussion, a source of great information and willing ally in exploring the non-consensual world.

I feel an enormous gratitude for the partnership with my editor Patricia Hoyle. We worked closely from the book's inception: her positive words and ability to extract the gold from my first scribblings encouraged me to keep going. Patricia also felt that we had to cooperate with something larger than we were. Finding that she too could not work in the normal linear set-yourself-a-goal-and-work-to-it fashion she said early on "this book won't be rushed". *The Wild Genie* had us in her thrall! At times Patricia could do radical surgery on the text, but always held my voice. Her gentle questioning, her thoroughness to detail and instinctual feel, have helped to mature the text enormously.

I am deeply grateful to my many friends and colleagues who have hung in with me over the years helping me directly and indirectly. The following people gave much valuable feedback on the text: Julie Cunningham and Amrita Hobbs both gave a rigorous appraisal of the book which sharpened my ideas. It was Julie who picked up the term "the wild genie" from the text and urged me to use it as the title. An inspired recommendation! With Jen Fox I was also able to clarify ideas on power, the nature of the Feminine and soul life. Francesca Naish, a naturopath and well published author, was also endlessly patient around publishing details and health matters, giving information and encouragement. Naturopath Karin Cutter, and her assistant Katherine Mooney answered my endless health queries with great wisdom and equanimity. Amy Scully, my assistant on numerous workshops gave me valuable insights and much enthusiasm for this work. Jane Bennett, Felicity Oswell, Anthea Ellison, Penny Fenton and Shushan Movsessian all helped me to clarify the text and offered helpful information. Sandy West has been a quiet ally in the background with financial assistance should I have needed it. Knowing this was always available allowed my psyche to relax into the process of writing. With Caroline Davis, Margaret Bailitis and Susan Dickson I have shared many rich explorations of inner life, ideas on therapy and received quiet support for the, at times, lonely journey with my health and this book.

I am indebted to the work of Penelope Shuttle and Peter Redgrove, whose seminal book *The Wise Wound* I discovered in my twenties and was the first thing I wanted to reach for when my menstrual woes erupted in my early thirties. I knew it would hold keys to my suffering. Latterly, *Alchemy for Women: Personal Transformation Through Dreams and the Female Cycle* has given me valuable insights. The work of Lara Owen, *Her Blood is Gold* and *Honouring Menstruation: A Time of Self Renewal*, has been critical in helping me to deepen my appreciation of the inner life of women at menstruation. Through her friendship and writings I felt I could come closer to cherishing the female body and the vistas that it opened me to. Judy Grahn's provocative and compelling take on menstruation and culture in *Blood, Bread and Roses: How Menstruation Created the World* fired me and gave useful insights about taboo and power. While I did not draw directly from the work of Chris Knight and his wonderful book *Blood Relations, Menstruation and the Origins of Culture*, like all of the above literature, it formed a solid background from which I could draw support and inspiration as I stepped onto the path of my own ideas.

I found the writings of Robert Sardello on soul life electrifying which, along with the work of Nor Hall, propelled me into my own thrilling appreciation of what the Feminine is really about. My whole understanding of the menstrual world expanded. I am deeply indebted to Process Oriented Psychotherapy or Process Work, developed by Arnold Mindell, and to my teachers, Arnold and Amy Mindell, Max Schupbach and Julie Diamond, for my understanding of symptoms and their connection to the world. The inspiration from Process Work helped me to climb out of the deep hole of powerlessness I experienced from my health woes. I was introduced to the idea of liminal space and how to negotiate the line between the consensual and non-consensual world, which through their menstrual cycle women always need to do. I also learnt valuable skills for working with altered states.

Thank you to Joanne Arnold for seeding the original concept and design of the cover. Unfortunately due to circumstances beyond her control, she was unable to complete it. I am very grateful to Eri Jinaka for stepping in at the last minute to develop the final, stunning version.

To the many health practitioners who helped me heal my body over the years and help me to maintain my wellbeing today (you know who you are!) I feel enduring gratitude. Your patience and knowledge continue to deepen my understanding of the healing process.

I also thank my body — it is here that the book began! But for the vagaries of my health, I would never have picked up on the topic of menstruation. My body was my teacher, guiding me to something, and I, the somewhat reluctant student! I hope I have honoured the spirit that was urging me on. And I give thanks to it for I love where I find myself today.

Contents

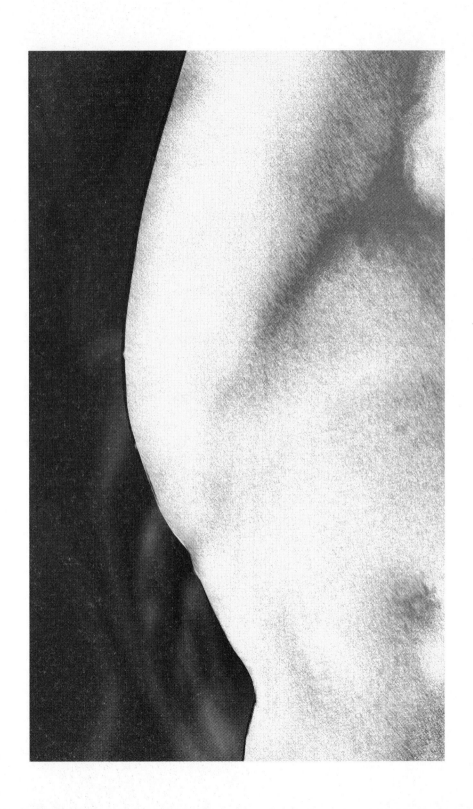

Revealing the Jewel

"THROUGH OUR MENSTRUAL EXPERIENCE WE ARE
EMBROIDERING OUR CREATIVITY. POWERFUL WOMEN
CREATING OURSELVES, CREATING THE WORLD."

Alexandra Pope

Revealing the Jewel

Women, menstruation and power

Menstruation is significant. In fact, it's loaded. In all my research into menstruation and menstrual health one theme burst through loud and clear: **power**. The power is present even in the word menstruation which, from the earliest cultures, also meant "incomprehensible", "supernatural", "sacred", "spirit", "deity" (Walker, 1983 p.635). In German, French and Spanish the word for menstruation also means "measure" or "rule" and connects with the terms regulate, regal, regalia, and *rex* (king). Terms that link menstruation to orderliness, ceremony, law, leadership, royalty, and measurement (Grahn, 1993).

The word "blessing" originates from the old English "bloedsen" which means bleeding. In Celtic Britain, claret was the traditional drink of kings. It was also a synonym for blood, and literally meant "enlightenment". According to the Taoist tradition in China a man could become immortal (or at least long lived) if he absorbed menstrual blood, called red yin juice, from a woman's Mysterious Gateway (Walker, 1983). The significance and power of menstruation, or as researcher and writer Barbara Walker describes it, "the spirit of sovereign authority" (p. 638), resonates loud and clear in many cultures across the world.

What secrets were they in touch with back then? What was it about menstruation that made it so loaded? Does this have any relevance for the 21st century woman? Does it have a connection with the menstrual disruption and suffering too many of us experience? And how could we use this power? I was intrigued.

In healing my own body I have tasted something of this power — and it's good! But I've learnt that it's not simply handed to us on a plate when we first start to bleed. No, we must grow into it. As few of us today have any appreciation of this potency, it's as though menstrual disturbance and suffering is one way this knowledge is being revealed to us, one way we can be inducted into this power. Our experiences of menstruation, which for many can be extreme, are uniting womb, heart and head. They are restoring and re-storying us and the world.

Our menstruating years give us the opportunity to hone our power. And menopause is our graduation day! The woman who has crossed the menopause having understood the power of her menstruating years is truly a woman to be reckoned with. She has been offered, through the dynamics of her own body, a way to travel in both inner and outer worlds. She has stoked a fire inside which is now brilliant, fierce, enduring. She can warm herself on it, be powered by it. A power that allows her to know and love herself and the world as one, and to act accordingly.

Is this book for you?

The Wild Genie presents a unique approach to menstruation that moves beyond biology to restore a dignity and deeper meaning to a woman's cyclical nature. This self empowerment is the most potent of elixirs. No herb, vitamin or drug is a replacement for a woman's discovery of her wisdom and strength. These are the qualities that are hidden within our menstrual experience — whether we suffer or not.

The Wild Genie is a self care guide for all women in their menstruating years who want to enjoy their cyclical nature and experience a long, fulfilling and healthy life — looking utterly gorgeous to the end! But if you're in, or beyond, the menopause you may want to take a peek over your menstruating sisters' shoulders for curiosity's sake. Perhaps to reflect and recover some knowledge that may ease your transition or deepen appreciation of the post menopause years.

This book is also for all parents who wish to pass on a positive experience of menstruation to their daughters and for men to help them gain insight into the world of women. If you're a man living with a woman who has a difficult time with her bleeding, you'll find lots of useful information that will help you to understand her better.

I wrote *The Wild Genie* because it was the kind of book I needed when I was in strife myself with extreme menstrual problems. I didn't want to take drugs or have surgery — and I was not keen to spend the rest of my menstruating years putting up with the menstrual pain from hell! I came to realise that no one health practitioner, including doctors, held the whole story. My healing was rooted always in my capacity to listen and respond to my body and myself — my self care. If I was to get well I was going to have to take responsibility and I became fascinated by all the things I could do for myself. I am now pain free. Menstruation has been utterly transformed for me, and I have been transformed by it. My hope is that you will become equally fascinated and transformed.

The ideas I present are not definitive, they are not a set of intractable rules. I offer you a different way of thinking about menstruation and your wellbeing so that you can expand your understanding. You may find my ideas sit just right with you. Or sometimes you may find yourself chaffing at what I say — if you do, I encourage you to ride with your own intuitions. Keep yourself open to the wisdom of your own being. For those of you who don't suffer from menstrual health problems, the information in this book will support your ongoing good health. Some of you will find the information enough to restore wellbeing while others will need to seek extra help from health professionals.

In my book I have focused on the underlying themes common to a range of different symptoms rather than referring to specific diseases, although I do sometimes mention conditions such as endometriosis, fibroids or Premenstrual Syndrome.

Through my writing I will help you reimagine your experience of menstruation. To imagine it's useful, positive and empowering. To allow the vitality of imagination to revivify yourself and the world. For those of you at odds with your menstruating body, or who suffer, it's possible to find peace and pleasure, and to heal, even in the face of apparently incontrovertible evidence. Even though you might still suffer from, let's say, bad period pain, it won't have the same debilitating hold on you if you can change your thinking about it. Imagination allows meaning to unfold thus altering your experience of the pain. What was once deeply disempowering, is now alive and powerful — even if it's still a difficult, recalcitrant power!

It's **your** particular experience of menstruation that will lead to meaning. By allowing yourself to go with the pain, distress or simply your experience of menstruation, you'll begin to find a way to the power. It's not always easy, particularly when your menstrual experience disrupts your work life, relationships and friendships. You may feel lonely and unloved because of your symptoms. I'm not disputing these realities. But if you're stuck in rage or resentment your suffering will be worse. You'll have both the pain, and the pain about the pain!

I will guide you to become curious, your own detective, to go to lots of different sources to gather information, to ask lots of questions until you're satisfied, and to go elsewhere if your health practitioner doesn't like this approach. Always remember that you're the one who has to live with your body — no one else! What might feel right for you may not look right to others. Consider carefully what others have to say. But always trust your own innate wisdom.

I will also help you to become difficult. This is my favourite! According to distinguished American surgeon Dr Bernie Siegel it's the "difficult" person who heals. The so-called problem patient is also the rapid healer, the long-term survivor, and the one with the active immune system (Siegel, 1988). The difficult person is the one who doesn't go along with the status quo, the one who is not "nice" at the expense of their own wellbeing. They are the catalysts for change in the world. They are difficult because they sometimes speak uncomfortable truths. Changing your diet, taking a fiercer stand for your needs, not always being there for others in the way they are used to may initially create discomfort for you and others. But that doesn't mean that what you're doing is wrong — it's just different. In this book I encourage you to make difficultness a high art — it's making you healthy!

As you embark on your healing journey I encourage you to give yourself Time. Slowness is fine. I've had many years acclimatising myself to this knowledge. There are some things I automatically do today that two or three years ago I would not have found easy. We have been seduced by the notion of instant results in everything, failing to value the necessity and beauty of Time in wroughting satisfying and lasting changes. Nature and our bodies need time. Speed prevents gentle observation and intimacy ... with ourselves and with others. Some of the information in this book will not sit easily in a hectic schedule.

More often than not our symptoms are urging us to slow down or do something different. And you may surprise yourself by how quickly healing occurs when you adopt some simple thoughtful remedies.

A word about symptoms

We're **not** meant to suffer when we bleed. Our menstrual suffering, that's so often passed off as "normal", is neither normal nor our lot. The menstrual cycle is the stress sensitive system in women. When we experience distressing symptoms, it's a signal to attend to our overall health and place in the world. Illness and physical symptoms are like signals leading us to new ground: under ground, above ground, into the world, lots of places. Illness opens the way. It's "the irrepressible imagination breaking through our adapted mediocrity" (Hillman and Ventura, 1992, p. 155). Menstrual distress is like a wild disturbing genie that has come to shake up this "adapted mediocrity". Imagination bursting her traces! We can try jamming the genie back in the bottle by denying these energies in us, and by colluding with a culture that says these symptoms are definitely an irrationality that need curing. But the genie will continue to wriggle and squirm.

The word healing can mean many things: recovery from illness; no longer experiencing uncomfortable symptoms; feeling more at peace with who we are; feeling that our life is meaningful even in the face of suffering; feeling empowered. Inevitably, healing involves exploration into many different areas, from the physical to the spiritual. Menstrual difficulties, like any other health problems, are linked to many factors including poor diet; overweight or underweight; poor digestion and immune system; hormonal imbalance; congenital and hereditary weaknesses; over-stressed life; personal psychological trauma; environmental pollution; low self esteem; cultural devaluation of the feminine; and, unbalanced energy systems.

These are all interconnected. A poor diet will depress your immune system, as will stress. Your hormones can be out of balance from too much stress, a polluted environment or poor diet. Low self esteem can be party to stress. And you can feel bad about yourself just because you're unwell or live or work in a discriminatory environment. They're all fundamental to your healing. And when you begin to heal one of these areas you will be led to the others.

Arnold Mindell, the originator of Process Oriented Psychotherapy, believes that illness does not happen in isolation, it's not the individual's "problem". Those who suffer are the canaries in the mineshaft alerting us **all** to danger and the need for change. Their increased sensitivity illuminates the landscape of everyone's lives. To put the onus of healing onto the individual deprives us all of vital information. Although suffering does have individual meaning, and there is an individual responsibility to attend to that, your illness does not mean you have personally failed. You're part of the great stream of life. Your individual difficulties mirror the times you live in — what happens in the world is everyone's responsibility. Inherent in your suffering is the voice of the activist, the initiator of change. Whatever positive steps we take for ourselves can become a gift for everyone.

When we're unsuccessful in our healing, whether we try orthodox or alternative approaches, we may feel a sense of personal failure, that it's our fault. We think, or are told, that if only we were more in touch with our feelings, more together, more balanced, more aware we wouldn't be sick. Such thinking doesn't make for good medicine.

Health practitioners can also get frustrated when their

treatment doesn't seem to be working and might imply that the fault lies with some failing on the part of the patient. Although you do need to attend to things yourself, it's important not to feel tyrannised. A good practitioner will have the wisdom to appreciate the complexities of each individual's journey.

I recognise that healing can be financially draining. The cost of regular visits to health practitioners and the various remedies such as herbs, homoeopathics, vitamins and minerals can become exorbitant over a period of time. Eating well is also expensive. But to cut corners with your health is false economy if you're spending lavishly in other areas of your life. I encourage you to simply do the best you can according to your budget. Regard your health spending as an investment — with good health other things will flow, including your ability to increase your income.

Some of the health care practices I recommend in this book have not been scientifically researched and therefore are not "proven". Yet, if I had waited for scientific research to come up with the answers, I would still be in pain. It's also not clear why some orthodox approaches are effective, yet we continue to use them. There are many instances today and in medical history where actions have been taken based on unproved evidence. For example, in 1845 a young Viennese doctor, Ignace Semmelweiss, discovered that handwashing before carrying out pelvic examinations of women in labor prevented "child-bed fever", infections that could lead to death. Semmelweiss' superiors objected to his "unscientific anecdotal observations" and fired him. His hypothesis was rejected by the medical establishment for over twenty-five years, yet today washing hands is the most basic infection control practice (Crook, 1986).

Menstrual problems are not generally life threatening — although they can certainly be "quality of life" threatening. The promises of orthodox medicine can be seductive and some women do find drugs and surgery necessary at times. However, orthodox medicine often assumes a single cause for illness, and that all individuals suffering from a particular disease are similar — so similar remedies are prescribed. In reality menstrual symptoms, and experiences of diseases such as endometriosis, are many and varied.

The doctor can cut a heroic figure, like the knight in shining armour sweeping us out of the nasty place to live happily ever after. Oh, that this were really so! The difficulty is what happens the other side of the sunset — the Next Day and the one after that and the one after that. Life after being "saved". Surgery may remove the offending fibroid, temporarily ease the agonising symptoms of endometriosis; and drugs may knock out the awful pain, smooth out the emotional moodiness, all of which may be necessary. But there's often a price to pay for engaging the body in aggressive health care approaches.

Surgery and drugs carry risks and side effects and may only temporarily resolve the problem. You're still left with the same body — will it produce another fibroid, rebuild the endometriosis? Quite possibly. Described as weapons in a war against disease, drugs are strong and toxic. As Dr Andrew Weill, a Harvard trained physician points out these suppressive treatments may actually strengthen disease processes rather than resolve them (Weill, 1995). Even if you do choose surgery and drugs, they're not a long term substitute for your own self care. Give thanks that they exist, use them judiciously and continue to support your body to heal itself.

Taking painkillers, or being on the Pill, may be how you've coped in the past — the idea of being without them probably sounds horrifying. I'm not recommending that you throw them out. But keep the painkillers for emergencies and start following the ideas in this book. If you're taking the Pill, or one of the medications prescribed for endometriosis, and would like to stop, make sure you're fully informed of the alternatives and keep taking the drugs while you're putting the appropriate alternatives in place. You need to discuss with your health practitioner all the choices you're making, or wish to make. Come off the drugs when you're ready and in consultation with your health practitioner — only change to something that genuinely supports you.

I have always felt that unsettling experiences, and in particular our menstrual disburbances, are like the dancing lessons of life — instructions from the Goddess, continually pulling us in, nudging us along, constraining us to the one path that is ours and ours alone. Your challenge is to relish the beauty and strength of that path that is yours, to dare to reveal it to the world. My desire is that this book will help you do this.

Finding your way

The first part of *The Wild Genie*, **Restoring Imagination**, tells the stories of three women, including my own. Stories that illustrate the themes of this book: women using the menstrual experience as a way to restore dignity and meaning to their lives, to discover an expanded understanding of female power, and to heal and love themselves. **Initiation**, explores menstruation as a time of power, the nature of that power and the value of cyclicity. In **Listening to Yourself**, I explore the range of recognisable premenstrual and menstrual symptoms, and show you how to transform the powerlessness of this suffering into something meaningful and a strength to heal. You'll discover how menstrual symptoms point the way to a greater understanding of the deep feminine and female power, both acutely needed in the world today. In **Using the Power of Menstruation**, I explore ways for you to relish your bleeding and heal your symptoms by attending to your soul and body. Simple and clear guidelines about what foods are supportive and unsupportive for healing menstrual difficulties and maintaining wellbeing are set out in **Nourishing Your Body. Menstruation, The World and You**, explores how you can manage commitments to others without jeopardising your own needs during the menstrual phase. And I guide you to recognise and value how your own individual cyclical tendencies and healing practices benefit the whole community. In **Down to Earth** you'll find useful reminders, recipes, home remedies and a variety of health care practices to enhance your menstrual wellbeing. **Finding Extra Help** lists practitioners, organisations, support groups and healthy products. If you're interested in reading more widely, you'll find a valuable list of books in **References** and **Further Reading**.

I encourage you to read through the entire book in sequence. Ruminate on its contents and notice what catches your attention, what makes the most sense to you. You might find yourself saying "Yes!", albeit sometimes tentatively to some ideas, or curling up and saying "Oh, no, that feels too much" to others. Go with the "Yes" — you'll be more motivated which means you'll have more success. And each success will encourage you to take another step.

Restoring Imagination

"IMAGINATION SERVES AS A
HOMOEOPATHIC ELIXIR THAT HEALS"

Robert Sardello

1. *From Pain to Power —* *My Own Healing Journey*

The pain hit just before my thirty-first birthday, a challenging gift from my body. And the beginning of my long journey of healing menstrual problems, fatigue and allergies. Although painful, this experience transformed my life and introduced me to a new passion and aspect of my career.

Fatigue was the only striking health problem during my twenties. I also suffered from allergies due to environmental factors but I had become so used to these I didn't think of them as ill health. Having a fierce will, I would let nothing stand in my path! I kept pushing and pushing myself until, in January 1984, my body dreamed up "the menstrual pain from hell". Now **that** made me stop and pay attention!

The pain each period was persistent, unrelenting. It could last for up to four days with varying intensity, the third and fourth days being the worst. All I could do was stop and journey with my body through the pain. This could take up to six hours and forced me to take to my bed. Over time, I was able to reduce the pain of the first and second days of the cycle — that general crampy, all over yukkiness, the heavy and aching feeling. The third and fourth day were another story altogether.

On day three I would wake feeling fairly clear of the general crampy stuff. And then suddenly around 10.30 in the morning — it was that precise — I would feel a faint shudder go through me, a slight heat. I knew the other pain had begun. It would take about two hours to build, coming in waves, small at first, but growing in a crescendo of agony. It felt as though something wanted to get out of my body, as if I was having labour pains. Between each wave there was a brief respite and then another mind numbing surge of it. They would come closer and closer together. Sometimes I would vomit. Other times I had diarrhoea. Although I have never given birth, I have it on good authority from women who have had children and experienced extreme menstrual pain that it can be as bad, or worse, than labour pains.

I felt as though I was being tossed around at sea in the wildest of storms — only to be dumped unceremoniously on the ocean shore when the pain stopped. I chose, wherever possible, not to take painkillers — the pain at its worst actually made a mockery of any painkiller. This was a mega force I was dealing with, not to be silenced by a puny little tablet! I screamed and rocked because this seemed to ease things, if only psychologically.

There was a point at which the pain would peak and then start to diminish, the waves getting smaller and smaller until finally they eased at around 3.30pm. I would slip into what felt like a drugged sleep for an hour or so. During the worst times, in my early thirties, the pain could even revisit on the fourth day, if I was not meticulous about diet. But generally the end of this pain signalled the end of the agony for that month.

After the pain had passed I would feel extreme exhaustion. But also newly born and slightly euphoric, probably high on my own endorphins, the body's natural painkillers, which get released when you're in pain. But despite this renewal of spirit, my physical energy sometimes did not pick up again until I ovulated, so challenging to my body was the pain experience.

Like many women, I was given the loud and clear message that menstruation was something to ignore as much as possible — get on with life, nothing is different. To reveal any suffering or difference at "that time of the month" was a sign of weakness, even a betrayal of women.

Nevertheless, I consulted a doctor, who suspected endometriosis and arranged an ultra sound. This revealed nothing abnormal. The next step was a laparoscopy, which involves a general anaesthetic and making a small incision in the abdomen to allow the surgeon to view the pelvis through a camera (laparoscope). I was not keen to have any surgery — however small the incision. When I asked my doctor, who was aware I would not take drugs, "If I get a name for what's happening, will it make any difference to the treatment?" she said "No".

So I said "No" to the surgery, skipped getting a name for my disease and decided to chart my own course of healing. I'm enormously grateful to this doctor, who respected my approach and made sensible suggestions, such as a particular type of stomach massage that increased peristalsis and gave me wonderful bowel movements, which in turn eased my pain. This was the first clue that the state of my digestive system was connected with my menstrual pain.

Living in Japan in my early twenties I had studied the beautiful, and sometimes physically demanding, movement discipline Shintaido. Shintaido has its roots in traditional martial arts but is equally at home within the arts, particularly with more avant garde forms of dance, theatre and music. I mixed with wonderful people, Japanese as well as foreigners, who exposed me to radical ways of viewing and experiencing the world.

Although it did exhaust my body, my training in Shintaido gave me a discipline and willingness to face difficult things without running away. Through this discipline I also experienced transcendent and ecstatic states — just remembering them now moves me. I learnt about altered realities and had deeply spiritual moments.

I took the Pill briefly, while in Japan, for contraceptive purposes. I thought it a Good Thing ... women's sexual freedom and all that. But it was a shallow victory. At the time I was blessed with an enlightened Japanese boyfriend who felt it was wrong to manipulate my body in that way. He wasn't interested in getting me pregnant — he was simply concerned for my wellbeing and was willing to do his bit to prevent conception. To this day I am very grateful to him — it helped me realise that my body didn't, and still doesn't, tolerate drugs well.

My experiences in Japan helped me to step outside the traditional medical model to embrace a far wider story for my suffering body. I would never have achieved the wellbeing I experience today if I had stayed within the boundaries of Western medical orthodoxy.

But when my pain first erupted 17 years ago, there was little information on alternative approaches to menstrual health. I felt as though I was inventing the wheel with my healing. I began with shiatsu massage and a very strict macrobiotic diet, an oriental approach to food. Having been introduced to this in Japan six years before meant it didn't feel strange to me.

Miraculously, after three cycles, suddenly no pain! But alas, this was not to last. Not because the diet didn't work but because I found it impossible to continue to follow it so religiously. It was as if my body needed me to know more about menstruation.

Also, I had to deal with the real world — I didn't do my healing in some mountain hut far removed from the vicissitudes of daily living. I was right in it. Living in a polluted city. Struggling to earn a living, studying, having relationships, dealing with the ending of those relationships. The usual wear and tear of daily life! Stress has an enormous impact on wellbeing and I had a fair dose of it. Diet alone wasn't going to cure that!

Gradually I came to learn that the menstrual pain was a signal of overall ill health. And only dealing with the menstrual pain wasn't going to fix things. I was constantly fatigued, had very poor digestion, suffered from allergies and frequently came down with colds and the flu. A classic story. My immune system was not a happy one.

I worked with an array of alternative therapies, in particular Traditional Chinese Medicine (acupuncture and Chinese herbs). I was so depleted it felt my acupuncturist brought me back from the dead. Healing takes time and I worked with him over a number of years — I am still grateful for his unending patience and care.

I discovered that no one health practitioner had all the answers. That was no failing on their part. No one has the whole story, this book included! The bedrock of my healing was attention to self care. The acupuncture, herbs, or whatever else I used, complemented this self care. I don't believe I would have overcome my health problems with the therapies alone. Initially my symptoms were so extreme, self care alone would also not have been enough although now I do find it usually maintains my wellbeing.

Yet, in all the valuable support and useful information I received, no one could give me a positive model of menstruation. Because doctors are generally only trained in the biological aspects of menstruation I did not expect to hear a positive view from them. Yet, perhaps unfairly, I did expect more from alternative health practitioners. But alas, the general feeling was that menstruation was a liability, something we just have to live with. Or even worse, that my suffering was because I was not in touch with my feminine nature. Remarks such as these made me feel judged.

The general feeling of negativity and judgment around menstruation bothered me. How could my body be well in such a climate? I needed an ally, so I began to see a psychotherapist to help me take a stand for these experiences. As a psychotherapist myself, I have always worked with psychotherapy models that embrace illness, or the problem, with curiosity and enormous respect rather than as an offending sickness to be removed. In a holistic approach the symptom is a signal you need to listen to and attend to, rather than something that should be cut out or removed without exploring the deeper story behind it. My psychotherapist helped me to look at my menstrual problems in this light.

We used imagination. We explored through my dreams, visualisation, play, poetry and metaphor. It was as though my menstrual process was peopled with characters. A turning point came when one day I turned up for my session in my premenstruum, about to bleed. By this time I had honed my skills in attention to myself and self care at menstruation. Like a Zen Buddhist monk I could handle the solitude and focus required. My therapist looked me squarely in the eye, "You know all about this monk figure, you have no difficulty with the discipline of healing, I want to know about the figure at the heart of your pain".

When I bled I slipped into another world ... a primeval delirium, the wild chaos of my pain. I roared. I had the abandonment of someone loosened by one too many drinks. Everything about my life fell into sharper focus. It was as though for a brief moment I was allowed to "see into" things. A moment of privileged access, a curtain being drawn back, only to close once the pain receded.

Through my pain I experienced such a strong force. This force was an ancient powerful woman who made me examine who I was, what I was doing and how I might be letting myself down. She was unremitting in her gaze. I felt naked. She was the kind of wild woman who in polite society is locked away.

She has no care for social norms. Life ripples through her like an ecstatic force. I find her beautiful and terrifying all at once and I can only let her out in small doses. To understand and use her passion is a lifetime's work.

While I was seeing my therapist, I had a dream of a very old "bag lady", who had alighted on a bus. The passengers recoiled from her smell of poverty and street living. She was inured to this recoil and seemed in a state of bliss with an almost childlike smile on her face. She walked down the bus blowing a blue mist over the passengers so that the whole atmosphere of the bus took on a bluish glow.

Like the bag lady of my dream with her blue mist, I was blowing imagination back into my body. Restoring an important mystery which helped to re-empower me in the face of continued suffering. My body became a challenging teacher rather than the enemy. I felt a dignity in my experience of illness and pain, realising that it might contain something useful after all. I felt myself being transformed. And this helped me ride the continuing suffering. This process of restoring imagination is at the heart of my work with women, as a psychotherapist and educator, today.

At the beginning the journey felt endless. Countless trips to the various natural therapists. A fierce discipline to diet. Vigilant structuring of my time so that I was prepared for the disruption of menstruation — I couldn't maintain my normal schedule at all. Being partly, and later fully, self employed, gave me some degree of flexibility. I make no bones about the fact my life was greatly circumscribed. It was a lonely, humbling process. Dragged as I was into the very core of the darkest part of my being I learned patience and became a stronger and more resilient person.

The waves of pain I experienced on day three proved the most intractable. I could reduce their intensity but the action of the waves was always there. It was not until I did a particular type of bodywork that I had an incredible breakthrough — my "miracle" story. I worked with a woman called Zoee Crowley, a trained nurse and practitioner of a form of body work called orthobionomy. Zoee comes to Australia twice a year from Hawaii to teach and offer private sessions. I had my first session with her when I was 40, nine years after I first experienced extreme pain.

Orthobionomy is very subtle work but deeply relaxing, and, like homoeopathy, treats like with like. The practitioner amplifies what the body is already doing and this releases the particular tension. The significant ingredient to my initial session was the very particular work Zoee did on my pelvic area, including an intravaginal process, during which she worked on the tissues, ligaments and muscles, allowing the uterus to rebalance. I had already been told by a health practitioner that I had a prolapsed uterus — a uterus not in the position it's supposed to be. Zoee also sensed this as she worked with me.

This session occurred on the day my period was to begin, two days on I was to be sitting on a long haul flight to Tokyo. What had possessed me to book a flight on the third day of my cycle? I was horrified when I realised what I had done but it was too late to change. I, who was usually so organised around matters to do with my period, found myself on a plane anxiously looking at my watch acutely aware of the peculiar precision timing of this process. Nothing happened. Nothing kept happening all the way to Tokyo. Nothing kept happening on that third day for the next two cycles.

And then the pain began to creep back. Zoee was back in Australia six months after her last visit and I was lining up to see her! After my second session with her the same thing happened. I could maintain her "adjustments" for just so long

— then the pain would return. A chiropractor later worked extensively on me and told me my flat feet were affecting the pelvic region which was "jammed up". So I got orthotics to address this and finally Zoee's adjustments held. I feel an enormous physical strength in my pelvis now, I don't even always wear the orthotics.

I also researched for months the negative health consequences of dental amalgam. The information was compelling yet I hesitated making the decision to have my amalgam fillings removed, a lengthy, very expensive and potentially dangerous procedure. Then one-middle-of-the-night-alone-moment the absolute certainty that I must do it rose from my being. I couldn't get started fast enough and six weeks later it was done. Before I made the decision I had very positive dreams about my dentist. In one dream he was providing a home for distressed wild animals. That was certainly me: distressed and definitely wild. After the work was complete I had another extraordinary dream depicting the amalgam as creating energy circuits in my body. Any healing I received would get locked into those circuits, unable to reach the whole of my body. With the amalgam removed healing could be total. I was left with no doubt that I had made the right decision.

After I had left the worst of the pain behind me I still felt a great deal of discomfort and tenderness with the bleeding. It felt like the pressure of wind trapped in my body, and indeed passing wind eased the discomfort. Until my mid forties I still felt an extraordinary fatigue following my period. Now, while I still need to be careful to conserve energy, I feel so much sturdier.

Throughout much of my healing I had the support of an enormously caring partner. He would just hold and rock with me when I was in the worst of the pain, even when I screamed and cursed. Sickness can feel like an extremely isolating and meaningless experience. His companionship was a healing salve and helped me to deal with the isolation. The way he conducted his own life encouraged me to follow my body processes, to question and probe them, rather than fight them.

Through my healing I have come to love my cycle. It's like a secret activity in me which opens and shuts doors, gives fleeting glimpses of Other Worlds, sometimes allows me to flit through, takes me off somewhere else while to all the world I look perfectly normal! Sometimes it reminds me of the seagulls riding the shifts in air currents on the seashore near my home. I'm aware of the shifting atmospheres inside myself and adjust accordingly. These inner movements help me appreciate subtleties, train me in complexity and remind me that life is change. If I lose touch with my cyclical nature I start to feel that life has a certain "sameness" about it.

Now, in the first half of my cycle I feel like a young girl, fresh, somewhat innocent and open. In the past I used to feel like a new born foal — all legs and jerky new life, darting off, losing balance. As I have become stronger this uncoordinated creature has been replaced by the more self assured young woman. In the ovulatory space of the cycle she gives way to a competent woman, skilful at acting in the world and experiencing an easy happiness. It's a good space — worthy and positive. Yet something is missing. If I were to remain in that world I would soon become an empty shell — beautifully formed on the outside, functional, but at the same time empty.

When I fully enter the second half of the cycle I find what I am looking for — a complexity and impassioned power. I become a more fully formed woman — in touch with the dark as well as the light side of my personality. Layers and layers have been added to my being. I know too much and am unable to use it or don't know how to use it. A force takes over, particularly as the period comes closer. Yet my will is stronger, I can get things done. I can tackle demanding tasks and take on difficult people. I cut to the chase. I'll write this book assiduously. I can be picky, critical, less sensitive to others, more fully engaged. My naivete at ovulation becomes replaced by a hard boiled realism.

A dreamy meditative state also comes over me in the two or three days before I bleed. I am much more fascinated by everything around me. This becomes particularly acute into the first day or so of bleeding. If I have many tasks to do, particularly if they involve driving, I can get a headache unless I go slowly allowing for the dreaminess.

I also feel an acute sensitivity. A sensitivity to something that I can't name or see. It's as though, metaphorically, the ground under me starts to give. I no longer feel solid. I feel seen through and self conscious. Just before the blood is due, and if I am out socialising, I will suddenly become distracted, completely uninterested in what's around me. I want to go home but have no "sensible" reason for leaving — I have nothing particular I have to do. But my psyche has its own requirements that my mind is not always privy to. I have learnt to honour and value these requirements. And without fail, the blood arrives next day. For me, menstruation demands solitude.

My cycle doesn't always follow a neat order — it depends on what's going on in my life. Some months are more intense than others, sometimes fractured, other times incredibly loving and complete. Sometimes the world conspires to give me a mountain of work that I must do while I dream of soft beds and drifting. Instead I must surrender to the work I have to do, but moving at a slower, more reflective, pace. What is always apparent is the contradictory and even unpredictable quality of the cycle. I like the charge and depth of the premenstrual world but perhaps would not want to remain there forever. What nourishes me is the very fact of my changing nature and what experiences it opens me to.

I've always felt a natural high as the blood flows, a glowingness. But in recent times this has been amplified and can begin 24 hours before I bleed. These days I slip into a very silent, resonant territory. Like going into a church or great cave. I'm sometimes flooded by deep feelings of love, as though I were in love with someone. It's wonderful. Once the bleeding has begun I want to drop my bundle and drift. If I don't need to work, I can really go with this ... swimming in a sea of feeling and ideas. Not grabbing at anything. Time slows down and I feel plugged into the very centre of the earth, flooded with the numinous, with ideas and countless inspirations. It's vitally important I don't feel pressured so that I can reap from the depths of this time. If I don't experience these things I often feel incomplete, cheated of something.

Working doesn't necessarily completely preclude me from entering this territory as long as I minimise things as much as possible. My particular type of work as a psychotherapist lends itself to the sense of the sacred and intimacy of menstruation. But wherever possible I do try to avoid being too public, such as running workshops, giving lectures or speaking to the media. I once had to do a small piece about menstruation for television which was to be prerecorded at my home, on the first day of my period, as it turned out. I feel super daggy when I bleed and dressing up is the last thing on my mind. But on this occasion I had to look gorgeous and entertain a mini TV crew of three men wanting 10 second snappy original grabs. My dreamy menstrual mind rebelled. While I could have happily yarned on about menstruation until the cows came home, I felt speechless in the face of the program's demands. The men were very sweet and respectful and we played and laughed until we finally got something they were satisfied with. I was not less competent because I was bleeding, my psyche simply did not want to engage with what felt like superficial responses — the needs of my being and the needs of this program clashed.

As the bleeding draws to a close I enter a phase for a day or so of extraordinary clarity. It's as though the release of the blood clears the cobwebs and blocked tensions, creating an open space. Then around day 5 or 6 I dip, as if momentarily grieving for the sweet intimacy and deep sense of connection with life that's so intensely amplified as I bleed. Soon after I'm picked up by the movement toward ovulation that leads me outwards.

My experience of menstruation has evolved over time. Each month I continue my initiation. My cycle and my period, like life itself, is changeable. A highly sensitive monitor for my life. I could switch off to the subtleties by not changing the rhythm of my outer life. But I suspect I would be revisited by a terrible greyness, and the fatigue and ill health I used to experience.

To heal I needed to restore imagination to my body. I was deeply grateful to my therapist for being the catalyst to open me to my deep and, what felt to me, dangerous regions. My menstrual pain gave me a lesson in power, a power connected with the Deep Feminine. It taught me to trust the authority of my body/being through instinct, intuition and dream, critical for me in unfolding the appropriate path to health.

I also realised I had to leave the confines of my monk's cell — I had to become a social activist. I learnt that my symptoms were an awakening, not a personal failing. They revealed to me something of the atmosphere of the society in which I lived. They demanded that I challenge those unsustaining ideas and practices.

My experience of pain stripped back the artificial elements in my life. It made me more honest. The qualities that I encountered through my pain are those least valued by my culture which loves order, logic, straight lines, setting goals, working hard and being productive. Through my pain I encountered myth, chaos, spirals, dreams, feelings and ecstasy.

My private healing became public. The more I researched menstruation, whether in mythology, ethnograpy, cultural studies or medically, the more convinced I became that menstruation wasn't the core problem. My menstrual problems were in part the symptoms of a culture that had a limiting view of menstruation. A culture ill at ease with difference, in particular anything to do with women. I realised that if women could validate their experience of themselves and ride with their changing nature, their whole experience of menstruation could be changed. And, most importantly, their suffering decreased.

The influence of environmental pollution on health, the difficulty of accessing good quality food, clean air and water became increasingly clear to me. I realised that, despite a public health system in Australia, health is a privilege. Doctors and hospitals can do little to make sure you have a good enough income to afford quality food, live in a healthy environment and have clean water and air.

Each month I marvel at how my suffering has lifted. I'm left now only with the pleasures of menstruation. It has taken years for me to reach this point. It has felt like forever. Whether you are suffering or not, my hope is that through my own suffering I will teach you to value the language of your beautiful, powerful body.

2. From Darkness to Discovery — Janice's Story

A passionate and bold woman, since her early life Janice has always felt an inordinant power surge through her. Although she has a strong intellect which has served her well, it was menstruation that taught her to use her power wisely. It taught her about the intelligence of her body and helped her find her true path.

Dux of her school in Year 10, Janice was an outspoken young woman, always ready to stand up against injustice, and in her own words, "on the road to being a lawyer or actor". Otherwise a healthy teenager, Janice suffered from extreme pain from her very first period. Her doctor told her that when she had children the pain would go. She "knew" she would never have children and felt abandoned by the medical profession. She believed the pain was a curse for not wanting to have children.

At 16 Janice's life changed profoundly. She saw the movie "Carrie" and thought it was "a stupid Stephen King film, but I knew there was something significant about it." The film is about a young girl who develops telekinetic skills — she can move objects without touching them — which are triggered by her menstruation. The morning after watching the movie, Janice woke up with a temperature. She couldn't walk and she had lost her sense of touch.

Doctors were convinced she had meningitis. But all the tests were normal. Her temperature came down but she still couldn't walk. In hospital she was placed in a room on her own and the psychiatrist was sent for. Initially she didn't like him and wouldn't talk. For three weeks she was confined to bed or wheelchair and remained silent. After the first week of feeling paralysed, she knew she was able to walk, but wouldn't. To this day she still doesn't understand why she maintained her disengagement — she just did. "If I couldn't be powerful I'd be the opposite, weak. I was starting to become aware of myself as a strong woman, never interested in boys, rebellious. I was going to be the first Australian woman prime minister. I was a feminist and didn't know it!"

In hospital for a month, her school was informed that she was suffering from a mental illness. Although the school staff and students treated her kindly she still felt some shame. It was difficult for her not to feel like the skeleton in the family closet.

Adolescence can be a turbulent time, menarche potentially both thrilling and disturbing. There are many stories from different cultures that tell of girls having extreme power at this time. Those women who become shamans, or healers, assume their religious and medical functions at the menarche. They become wedded to the supernatural and "acquire the conversation" of the deities and guardian spirits. The Mojave girls are told that whatever they do or dream at this time has significance for their future. (Shuttle and Redgrove, 1989)

At 16 Janice had already been menstruating for a few years. Yet it was the Stephen King film about the powers of a young menstruating girl that she believes triggered her own powerful altered state. Was Janice afraid of the power budding in her and so turned away from it? What if her teenage "episode" was the body's dream that was giving her clues about herself and her future, even shaping her future? What if she were being alerted to pay attention in a deep psychic sense, to "other forces"? Losing herself in that moment was the beginning of a long initiatory journey of self discovery.

Her life changed — as though it had been completely rerouted. Dreams for the future completely fell away. After leaving school she didn't go to university and was more interested in partying — smoking, drinking and taking recreational drugs. Violent premenstrual anger burst onto the scene. Janice was at odds with the world. "I had an inkling all through my twenties that there was something I had to figure out. I never wanted children, was never good at relationships. Whatever life had in store it didn't hold babies and marriage. Am I gay? No. I've thought about it long and hard. I don't feel heterosexual either. I have a hard time convincing people I'm happy on my own. I'm strange … feel really different, trying to work it out and never finding an answer."

Spiralling into the depths Janice became caught in an internal battle of self loathing and rage played out in her wild behaviour and drug taking. Yet something in her maintained the line to an inner knowing. "Have a good time, Jan, get it out of your system," she would say to herself.

After working in women's housing, refuges and with incest survivors, she finally made it to university in her late twenties. She was drawn to politics and completed an honours degree in political science. She had found her path, her adolescent dreams for her life still intact, although perhaps not in the form that she originally imagined. Still a deeply committed activist, she is now setting her sights high in the world of policy and social reform.

When she finally made it to my therapy practice at 30 she had come a long way. But she needed to go deeper, to discover the meaning in it all and to heal her body. She was still experiencing severe period pain each month and premenstrual mood swings. Cranky with those around her she easily exploded, making her hard to live and work with in the few days before her period. As her story unfolded I quietly put my menstrual health notes aside. She was overweight, was binge eating and still smoking and drinking. Simply telling her to sort out her diet and stop drinking was hardly going to work. We needed to explore the stories driving her wild and uncontrollable behaviour.

At times I wove in information about menstruation. The incidents of binge eating gradually decreased and food has become much more manageable. Although the alcohol and cigarettes still figure they are greatly reduced. What's more important is that Janice is more self aware and respectful of herself. She can still feel rage although this is no longer locked into the premenstruum — her rage is less the enemy and more a power that she is learning to use rather than abuse.

We both feel her rage is not entirely personal, but rather fuelled by her deep feelings about social injustice. Now her anger informs her about where her work in the world lies. Although still there, her period pain is less intense, particularly when she takes care of herself. She commented once "Oh, I wish I bled every week I take such good care of myself around menstruation!" And menstruation for Janice is far from perfect. Yet she actually looks forward to the bleeding because "I give myself permission to go into that 'weird territory'. I lie in bed and roll around. I create the ambience of the cave with candles and beautiful things round me. The pain is bearable. It's worse if I have to consider anybody! The twinges tell me it's coming and I prepare. The right sheets on the bed, essential oils, and nice food in the fridge. It's a weird territory, it's almost as if I go into another plane of consciousness. It's like you're in this orb — your body sends out this invisible silken orb to rest in. And if you ignore the orb you bump into things and bruise. It's almost like amniotic fluid, returning to the womb. Women have the luxury of knowing about the womb. All the energy gets sucked into that part of me [the womb] and this helps with the pain. Women have been taught that knowledge worth knowing can't come from the body. And yet that's not so. I learn about my addictions, my hatred, pleasures, the way I react to work. Exploring those things in therapy I dovetail it with what comes from my cycle. Learning to understand the cycle has helped me to understand myself and it helps me to understand the world. It's helped me to understand my anger. It's such a journey. I'm learning to harness my power. I was a wreck when I turned up at therapy. I hated everything, I hated injustice. We were once burned [at the stake] for this power."

The pain for Janice has become a signal that helps her gather information about her health. And she uses her power thoughtfully in fighting the injustice that she hates. Now if Janice starts to feel a surge of anger in the premenstruum she asks herself: "What's going on, Jan?" She tries to be still so that she can find out what's triggering her anger. If she has been reactive she will apologise, without making the excuse that she is premenstrual. The premenstruum and menstruum used to be the murkiest phases for Janice — now they provide her with moments of real clarity. The key for her is not to pathologise her menstrual experience.

There's no doubt in my mind that the adolescent experience that changed her life so profoundly was a sign that she should take herself and her power seriously. She has always felt an outsider to some extent — in a tribal culture she might have been marked out as a person with "special powers". She would have received disciplined training so that she would neither abuse nor be abused by those powers. Instead she landed on the planet in the latter half of the twentieth century in a "modern" society where those particular types of talents often become pathologised. Without elders to train her she was left to wrestle alone in the dark with her particular talents.

Janice's initiation came after six years of hard study while she was finishing her honours degree. In the final week of writing her thesis she felt an enormous surge of power that drove her through those last few days to complete the work in time for the day of the deadline. She did it and that night her period came. For the first time in as long as she can remember she had almost no pain. In those last weeks her body was very neglected as she sat day and night writing — the pain should have been worse! When she told me the story we both felt a small frisson of energy. Although her menstrual pain has since returned, the completion of this thesis was the culmination of a long dream. It felt as though the lack of pain in that moment was a signal that she had honoured her soul demands. It was a rite of passage.

To be strong in the world a woman needs the capacity to love herself more than anything else. Menstruation has become a symbol of self care that is helping Janice value herself and undo her self loathing. Her capacity to take her own side, to look on her large body with increasing ease, and embrace her beauty, is growing. Through menstruation's disturbance Janice has learned to use her power wisely.

3. *From Chaos to Creativity — Amy's Story*

Within twelve months after her first period at 12½ Amy was menstruating every two weeks and would sometimes bleed ten days at a time. Not an auspicious beginning to her menstruating years and yet her menstrual disturbances became the catalyst for her journey into the feminine and her discovery of her artistic talents and psychic ability.

By age 14 she was already "pretty wiped out" by excessive bleeding so her doctor prescribed the Pill to help regulate her cycles. This at least made life more manageable, although later, when Amy became interested in boys, her mother told her in no uncertain terms it was "not a licence to have sex!"

Afflicted by a strange illness when she was 16, Amy found she had no energy. She frequently fainted and, not surprisingly, felt emotionally very low. She was diagnosed with a heart problem, mitral valve prolapse, and was treated for low blood pressure. Her illness, which lasted a few months, remained largely a mystery, even to her doctor.

The pain and heavy menstrual bleeding were waiting to greet Amy when she decided to come off the Pill at 17 although the period was at least slightly more regular, the cycle lasting for almost 4 weeks now. To Amy the pain felt like congested energy, which was more intense when she wore tampons. The fainting continued, often coinciding with her period or when she was in large crowds, and she had thrush and digestive problems much of the time. All was definitely not well with her body. Usually she coped by taking large quantities of painkillers, although on one occasion, when she was 20, the pain became so extreme she needed to be hospitalised and placed on a drip.

After leaving school at 16, she spent a year in business college, followed by a short course in cosmetics. She worked in a variety of responsible administrative positions and earned good money for her age. Wanting to be a businesswoman, to emulate her Dad, she worked hard, pushing herself.

At 21 it all came to an end. She left her job, her boyfriend and Sydney — the city she had lived in all her life — and moved to Melbourne. She wanted a change. Having grown up the youngest of a large family, she yearned to be away from everyone who knew her, to think and explore on her own.

It was the opening to an inner life, to her creative and healing talents. Soon after arriving in Melbourne, she also met her partner, Russell, with whom she now, at age 30, has two gorgeous, healthy children, Mimi and Marlon. She started a job but soon had to leave work because of her poor health. For the year that she wasn't working she had the space and time to engage with herself, listen to her body rhythms, get in touch with her dreams and even have out of body experiences.

She also started smoking and experimenting with recreational drugs — neither activity conducive to health — and began to have psychic and healing experiences. One night at a restaurant, she burnt her leg badly. The pain was so intense she was unable to sleep and wanted to go to the hospital. That night, Russell, her partner, encouraged her to breathe into the pain. She experienced a rush of heat into the area, the pain went away and she fell into a deep sleep.

Her menstrual pain, agony though it was, took on a kind of normality. Of course, the pain wasn't normal — but with so little public awareness around menstrual health issues and knowledge of genuine remedies for menstrual pain, it wasn't surprising she had learnt to accept and live with it.

But over the next three or four years, Amy's health problems intensified. She developed a cyst on one of her ovaries which burst in a nightclub one night, accompanied by a slight epileptic-like seizure, landing her once again in hospital. A laparoscopy revealed endometriosis — no further treatment was suggested so she resigned herself to continuing as before.

Creating small rituals, Amy also began drawing and learning about the Tarot, feeling a sense of familiarity with the cards. In her art she would find herself drawing what she called "lots of spirit figures", which intensified as she began the task of healing her menstrual problems.

After a trip to Nepal at 24, Amy had even worse stomach problems after contracting giardia. She felt drawn to doing rituals by the sea. This particularly helped her let go of "lots of stuff in the belly that I wanted to release" — a negativity and a stuckness that she wasn't able to name. Sometimes it felt like she was trying to reconnect "something that was severed in the laparoscopy". Like a reconsecration of her body. Her drawings were often of red raving women figures.

Then one New Year's Day, while staying at a beach house with friends, Amy was taken over by a ferocious pain. She was wearing a tampon which "was blocking everything", she said. "It was shocking. I was out there with the pain, there was nothing else going on for me except the pain. I was ravished by it and blacking out." This was a pain way beyond the reach of any painkiller. She thought she was dying, "I just wanted to go and lie down in the forest". Her friends managed to find a doctor a half hour drive away at a country hospital. The pain put her into an altered state so strong, she began to lose her sense of time. "Although I was in pain, I was in a bliss state. I thought this is it. I thought I was really going (to die) the pain was so bad". The hospital diagnosed a miscarriage. Amy was convinced it was not that, and felt even more distressed when the hospital staff did not take her seriously.

Following another laparoscopy, endometriosis was once again discovered. Her doctor indicated through drawings where the endometriosis had been — corresponding to all the places she had felt pain. Go back home to Sydney (where she and Russell were now living) and have a baby or hormone therapy, was the medical advice.

Early the next morning, still in hospital, a thoughtful and inspired nurse wheeled Amy onto the veranda to see the sunrise. "It was so beautiful — this was a sign, my wake up call to really look at myself."

Amy returned to Sydney, enrolled in art school and took herself off to healers in particular for acupuncture, Chinese herbs and regular shiatsu massage. She began a strict healing diet similar to the one I recommend in this book and finally received treatment for the giardia. Now a film make up artist, she also teaches film and theatre make up, including the use of masks, visualisation and ritual, to actors and designers. She also runs small Tarot groups with women and does Tarot readings.

In the midst of the extremes of the sickness, Amy had frightened herself. "I had the feeling that I wasn't earthed, that I was not in my body and that that was what was wrong. I wasn't happy with my home life or my work. I had no money." She needed to attend to all these elements. So she concentrated on grounding herself, going slowly, doing lots of walking and continuing her drawing and rituals. She also took up yoga and belly dancing and got a stable job. She was on the road to self healing. Everything began to ease: the clots, the pain — six months later she conceived her daughter, Mimi.

After the birth of her daughter the periods continued to

improve. Her mitral valve prolapse also healed. Amy now finds that her intense menstrual pain turns up as premenstrual rage — there's a force in her that will out! An intelligence, an inner knowing, maybe an ancient womanly knowing, that's recorded in the sinews of her being, in her feelings and struggles with her health. Although she's still learning to negotiate and harness this knowing, it's an intelligence born of deep self engagement. There are no short cuts, no slick techniques — only the continuing significant and sacred engagement with both the inner and the outer world.

Amy has an easy "witchy" talent, an ability to explore altered states (without drugs now!). In more woman-friendly times she might have been a temple priestess serving the divine feminine. Today she's learning to hold to that spirit in her enormously busy life as partner and mother as well as in the paid workforce. She continues to be fascinated by "the dark feminine stuff", by the "Goddess" and positive archetypes of powerful women.

Throughout the healing process, her partner Russell was very supportive. At that worst moment of New Year's Day he was terrified she would die and "really rode through it" with her. He always encouraged her creative expression as part of the ritual of her healing. Now that Amy no longer suffers the excruciating extremes of pain and can pay attention to menstruation by choice rather than out of necessity, Russell is ambivalent. It's a power he recognises as one that a man doesn't have access to and it makes him uneasy. "Intellectually, I'm OK with it. But at some really deep seated manly level, I'm fearful and in awe of it. I simply don't want to know about it. I'd really like it if she had a lodge up in the hills she could go to [when she bleeds]". Amy would love this too and curiously one of her dreams is to create a moonlodge, a place where women could gather when they bled. But both Amy and Russell contribute to the family income and like most families, their lives are complicated and busy. As long as neither of them runs from this tension at menstruation it will provide an opportunity for Russell to deepen his appreciation of the feminine and of women. In doing this their relationship will be deepened.

Amy came into my life just as she had conceived Marlon. As part of her exploration into "women's business" she wanted to learn about menstruation. She became my apprentice, assisting me at workshops and, in time, presenting segments of the sessions herself. Her sensitivity and ability to "see into things" helped me enormously to deepen my own understanding of this subject.

Today her whole cycle is distinct and clear. She knows exactly when she has entered the premenstruum. The fainting has long stopped and she is now consciously able to enter a trance state. If she isn't too overwhelmed by work, the day before her period can be a happy, "cruisy" time: peaceful, content and still. If she can't give enough space for her internal states then that moment can be marked by a headache. The pain, although greatly reduced, is still her companion. It's sometimes deep and sore but "if I can get quiet and still, I can release it. I can let it flow through me and that includes my head being in it. When I can lie and sleep and dream I can shift the premenstrual stuff too, but there's still that snappy raging energy."

No, that one doesn't want to be dreamt away — that energy's got business to be communicated out in the world! Her creativity, feyness and lightness of touch are combining with growing fierceness.

Initiation

At menarche a young woman enters her power, throughout her menstruating years she practises her power and at menopause she becomes her power.

Native American saying

1. *The Wild Genie*

What is it about menstruation that disturbs? What is it about our hormones, otherwise very well behaved and nicely turned out, that they should suddenly go wild on cue each month?

Menstruation is renowned for disturbing, the menstruating woman often the butt of innuendo, joke and ridicule. If it was only one or two of us suffering we might imagine it was some terrible personal flaw. But it isn't only one or two of us. Many women suffer at menstruation. Many keep quiet about that suffering. Women are even given the message that this suffering is normal and that we should just put up with it.

Think for a moment about society's messages about menstruation. Try talking about menstruation beyond the confines of one or two friends, try looking for stories about it as a positive, empowering experience for women. It's true there's a lot of medical information, orthodox and alternative, but the information is always about saving us from our "awful lot" of pain, PMS and lots of blood. Many of the ads on TV for tampons and pads buy into a mythology of "look normal", "pretend nothing is different", "no one will ever know" — keep that dangerous genie firmly in her place!

I'm curious as to what's so terrible about people knowing we're bleeding. In her magnificent book on menstruation *Blood, Bread and Roses: How Menstruation Created the World*, Judy Grahn describes the mystery of menstrual blood:

> *Menstrual blood is the only blood that is not traumatically induced. Yet in modern culture, this is the most hidden blood, the one so rarely spoken of and almost never seen, except*

privately by women, who shut themselves in a little room to quickly and in many cases disgustedly change their pads and tampons, wrapping the bloodied cotton so it won't be seen by others, wrinkling their faces at the odour, flushing or hiding the evidence away. Blood is everywhere, and yet the one, the only, the single name it has not publicly had for many centuries, is menstrual blood. Menstrual blood, like water, just flows (Grahn,1993, p.xviii)

Our collective discomfort around menstrual blood has its source partly in the excellent tutoring we've received in devaluing all that is female. But our loathing of the blood also speaks volumes about the fear of entering the deep world of female knowledge that lies in the experiences of the female body. It's as if our psyche senses this knowledge, but we don't want to know what the psyche knows. Because to know challenges the basis of how we conduct our lives. It could radically upset our apple cart and everyone else's too.

So each month as the "wicked genie" escapes from the bottle we go to doctors, desperately searching for a way to jam this wicked spirit firmly back in its place — forever. We are responding to a cultural message about menstruating bodies as something to be kept hidden at all costs. In turn, healers of all kinds are responding to our requests.

Yet the drugs we're offered to help us cope, such as the Pill, the many painkillers, and drugs for endometriosis, are a double-edged sword. Although bringing some very necessary relief, the side effects of some drugs border on the severe. Rather than healing the problem these drugs simply mask the symptoms.

Alternative therapies such as herbal medicine, homoeopathy, acupuncture and chiropractic have proved to be very successful with many women. Although these approaches look at underlying physical imbalances and any emotional difficulties, they still focus on illness as pathology without looking at the cultural and soul environment of the woman. For example, the menstrual pain may be treated successfully; however, the woman may still have little appreciation of how her illness can also be symptomatic of the culture she lives and works in. I experience this as part of the same conspiracy against the "wicked genie".

Something is definitely amiss. And I don't think we should keep quiet about it. This is not a private, individual affair — we're all colluding to silence this disturbing spirit. It's time to get curious about our wayward bodies! Something potent lurks there!

2.   *A Time of Power*

Reclaiming the feminine

The experience of powerlessness, fatigue and uncertainty is the best training in understanding their opposites. Female power, which has its source in the body, speaks through the body — menstruation's tendencies are the rich voices of the feminine consciousness.

Our menstrual symptoms are an entry point to power. Through our suffering, openness and vulnerability, we can gather our wisdom. But we don't have to be sick at menstruation to discover this. The process already exists, lying in the containment that the cycle provides — symptoms merely highlight the process. Within the crucible of our cycle we can gather the wisdom that's our power by riding the ebb and flow of the life of our body without manipulating or judging it, surrendering to the womb as she both creates life and allows us to recreate and renew ours each month.

I believe at menstruation, when our guard is down, we catch a glimpse of an old knowing, the power of the feminine. But because we have no validation for this experience we ignore it. The feminine has long been suppressed in both men and women. Yet it is women who have carried an inordinant amount of suffering for loss of Her. This instinctual and intuitive power, this soul voice, although given the poorest soil in the psyche to inhabit, is tough because of it.

I'm thinking of the Goddess in her many forms when I personify feminine consciousness as "Her". This is the same

Goddess that has been sacrificed to a male God. When I talk about "Her" I'm speaking of Her presence in both men and women. Rather than being "female" or "woman", She's simply an aspect of being human. When I refer to the masculine, I'm also referring to a way of being rather than to the male gender.

There are many aspects to the feminine. I notice my own awkwardness in approaching Her as though I'm still ill equipped to be writing about Her. Or is it I must come at Her in oblique ways, catch Her out of the corner of my eye, feel Her chaffing as I try to be too analytical? Analysis is not Her mode. She is not an "it" to be scrutinised. Rather She is to be experienced.

Traditionally the masculine is seen as the active shaper and the feminine the passive follower. We have largely internalised this as "active" equals power and therefore good, and "passivity" equals powerlessness and therefore bad. This has led to a gross misunderstanding, diminishment and distrust of the power of the feminine along with an inappropriate elevation of the masculine mode. To discount either the feminine or the masculine is to invite trouble. In Taoist China the female principle was seen as "active" and "creative" and the masculine as "passive" and "quiescent" (Walker, 1983).

True power comes from our ability to move fluidly between the two worlds of the masculine and feminine. But it's necessary to understand the distinctive nature of the feminine before we can know the whole.

The strength of menstruation lies in what we typically condemn in ourselves — our sensitivity. The amplification of our senses, amplifying our sense of the world. Our capacity to perceive through all our senses allows us to gather knowledge about the world without the filter of preconceived ideas. It's an "immediate knowing of things in their unity through the unity of the senses … Perception is a cognitive act of the body, knowing that is at the same time feeling." (Sardello, 1995, p. 176).

This is the feminine at work. Connection with the feminine frees us to receive the unknown coming to us from the future. It's not about letting go of what we already know but recognising that it is lodged in the past. In science, for example, major breakthroughs are often triggered by hunches, intuitions, and dreams (the feminine) which are later rigorously tested with the logic of the mind (the masculine). Logic itself cannot receive that breakthrough.

If we are to restore the power of the feminine we must also reclaim the language associated with it. Words and phrases like "being with", "letting go", "not doing", "yielding", "being moved by", "surrendering", "being guided by", "non-linear", "allowing", "being receptive". Inherent in these words is the knowledge that there is something beyond our small ego understanding of the world. A recognition of a relationship. A recognition of the world as a source, not a resource to be used for our own ends. This includes both the way we treat the Earth and each other. We are in relationship with everything. We are co creators, creating and being created.

Once we become open to this wonderful understanding we recognise that we're part of a living, breathing whole that can inform and support us. It's less tiring and more fun than always coming up with the goods all on our own. We have our own dreams and plans. At the same time we need to cooperate with and be touched by theworld which is alive with its own dreams and plans. It's this dynamic relationship between us and the Other which "is the crucible in which autonomy, creativity, compassion and wisdom are all forged" (Borysenko, 1996, p.25).

For me the experience of allowing and letting go requires enormous courage — it is a creative process and when I'm able to do so I'm filled with potency and activity. Perhaps this is what the Taoists meant when they spoke of the feminine principle as active and creative. While living in Japan I practised Shintaido, the Japanese movement art based on the martial arts, and also studied the martial arts of bokuto (use of the wooden sword) and bojitsu (use of a six foot staff). Through all these disciplines I learnt that the most powerful movement of all was the one where I looked the most vulnerable, the one which involved surrender and openness. It seemed to liberate both my "opponent" and myself.

Letting go allows the release of imagination — this is what truly gives life. The imagination fuels the physical activity. Activity without imagination is meaningless work. If the masculine has no knowledge of the power of His counterpart, the feminine, letting go is terrifying. It feels like loss of control, which we perceive as scary. Senior lecturer in English and Australian literature David Tacey, believes the feminine's "healing potions can look at first like poisons, and her wholeness can seem like a terrifying fragmentation to an ego that lacks the courage to accept her challenge." (Tacey, 1997, p. 173) When we live in a one sided world, the other side is experienced as dangerous or less valuable.

Imagination is like a prayer offered to the world. Instead of worrying about how to get what we want, imagination is like a magnet helping us find the way to realising our dreams. If we focus more on what we want than on how we're going to get it we're allowing the world to offer us something. This is co-creation at work.

I think I hear the masculine rattling His sabre right now, gesticulating to me. Telling me something about the importance of actually "doing things" — imagination is "all very well but would anything ever get done?". Well no — which is why we need the masculine as well.

The activity of the masculine principle is a wonderful capacity. But without the feminine's understanding of relationship and the interdependence of all life, He will act in ways that lack soul. Life becomes an activity without a deep encompassing intelligence — this leads to destruction. The feminine, without its partner, the masculine, can also destroy. But in the world today, I believe the masculine needs to learn a little respect for the "hidden" attributes of the feminine.

Failure to understand the feminine means being eternally set against the world. The world's speaking back to you will always seem an obstacle to be conquered rather than a necessary tension that's part of your evolution, or a guide that reveals.

To discover the feminine is to discover the Secret Garden: wild, verdant and changing. The nourisher of souls. Today we most often encounter Her presence, I believe, when we feel ill at ease, uncertain, limited and disturbed as we often do at menstruation. Although She is not these things, She speaks through them. The unease or disturbance allows knowledge of Her ways to come through. Intuition, instinct and ecstasy are some of Her modes. When you feel attracted to something, or want to stop, find yourself rebelling against what seems sensible, pursue the less well trod path, crave pleasure and long for the illumination of joy, you know you are honouring her ways.

She will not be discovered through control, rather She requires a relinquishing of that control. She's elusive, seemingly even perverse. She speaks the language of the heart. Our knowledge of the world will be forever half formed if we persist in only honouring the power of the mind, the logical masculine consciousness. Wisdom cannot take hold in a soil that lacks the moistness of feeling. Yet, resilient, She persists with us. She doesn't desert us even as we try to desert her. It is Her story that you will continually find at the heart of this book.

The element of danger

In all the many stories, myths and taboos surrounding menstruation there's the element of danger. Danger implies: "pay attention, wake up". A Yurok Indian woman speaking about menstrual laws handed down to her by her maternal aunts and grandmother, finished with the admonition that you should feel all of your body exactly as it is, and **pay attention** (my emphasis) (Buckley, 1988). There's something going on and if you don't stay awake not only will you miss it, you may get clobbered by it!

That's the nature of a taboo. The word "taboo" comes from the Polynesian tapua, meaning both sacred and menstruation. Besides sacred, "taboo" also means forbidding, valuable, wonderful, magic, terrible, frightening, and immutable law (Grahn, 1993).

Menstruation is a woman's inner wilderness territory. Native Americans regard menstruation as a woman's time of power because of her natural access to an expanded reality. The Native American practice of the vision quest — going alone into the wilderness — was traditionally the way men could enter a powerful limenal state to gather knowledge and seek visions and guidance. The ritual was particularly important to support young boys in their transition to manhood. Although women can also benefit from time in nature, it was believed that they did not need to challenge themselves in the same way in order to enter such a numinous experience. It would come to a woman unbidden as she menstruated. All she need do was be still.

A critical element in many initiation rituals for boys was to break their ego spirit — they must experience an ego death in order to enter the void. It was only then that they would come to understand that they're not self sufficient, that they need others for their survival (Tacey, 1999). It was their opening to the feminine.

Puberty rites for young girls emphasised education, celebration and strengthening of character. Any extreme practices had more to do with the particular culture's beliefs in menstruation's enormous power, power that had to be regulated by strict procedures so that it could not disturb the community. Girls did (and do) not require the severity of training that boys did (and do) because they had within their bodies, within the cycle itself, the process of induction. The menstrual transition shakes the ego — our very own built in monthly ego death. Loosening the boundaries, connecting us to the world.

The loss of control that happens at menstruation is, I suspect, the dangerous element for modern women. Instead of staying neatly in their box our emotions go walkabout at the slightest provocation — or even without it. Our body betrays us with spots, a bloated belly and pain. And I bet all those "bad hair days" and "none of my clothes fit" happen more often than not close to menstruation! Seemingly happy and comfortable with our lives we suddenly find ourselves questioning and doubting everything we ever did or do.

But what if we're meant to lose control a little? What if we're meant to question? What if this something lurking in our bodies is a quality women need more of in the world? A Good Thing that we only experience as a Bad Thing because it would be socially unacceptable to do otherwise? What if the disturbing mood swings, pain and other complicated symptoms were the result of not understanding the nature and usefulness of the menstrual cycle beyond its baby making function?

At menstruation we're being shaken up by something bigger than we are. Instead of fighting it, the proper response might be to allow ourselves to be opened and changed by saying, "I give up! I'm all yours, body! Where do you want to lead me?" The disturbance of menstruation provides an opening through which we can fall, like Alice falling down the rabbit hole, into a different reality. This reality may be frightening but it's not necessarily wrong.

Menstruation is meant to disturb. Disturbance in a system is a place of potential change and evolution because it makes us question and reflect. It's an essential ingredient for healthy democracy. We're meant to doubt a little, we're meant to have the axis of our life shifted. Such tension is a potentially creative moment. Our changing nature and disequilibrium is keeping us vibrantly alive. John Ralston Saul, a Canadian writer and social commentator, amusingly reminds us of the necessity for this: "On the day that you or I achieve a stable condition of equilibrium, those around us who have been less fortunate will draw one of two conclusions. Either that we are dead or that we have slipped into a state of clinically diagnosed delusion" (Saul, 1997, p. 158).

I'm not suggesting that women should put up with suffering, or abandon all remedies, whether conventional or alternative. But these medicines could be better used in the spirit of menstruation as a potentially empowering experience. One that gives us rich information about ourselves and the world. One for which a woman definitely should not be shamed or feel embarrassed about. If you are in extreme pain and can't feel a sense of empowerment, this is not your fault, as pain can obliterate other feelings. As you follow the suggestions in this book you may find your very distress is the doorway to the power I'm speaking of here.

Individuals experience different degrees of disturbance. Those more psychically, emotionally or physically sensitive may experience greater degrees of disturbance because of that sensitivity. This has nothing to do with failure or character weakness. It's actually providing information for creating wellbeing in ourselves and the world. Resistance to the disturbance is what amplifies suffering. By valuing our changing nature, not fighting it or seeing it as wrong, we can minimise the distress and turn it into something useful.

Menstruation becomes more hazardous if a woman fails to pay attention or take responsibility for her emerging self at this time. The danger signs we meet as we approach this land of bleeding are warning: "Tread with care because Power lurks here". Power can be dangerous if used without awareness. Unfortunately, Patriarchy has snuck in and doctored the warning signs. It has tried to re-route us altogether from this territory by telling us: "Ignore this space" or "Danger, keep away, this place is bad for your health!". But it's that very ignorance that's making us sick.

In our modern society we've dispensed with the stories of power, danger and magic. It's a power we're uneasy with, perhaps because menstruation is a uniquely woman's process. While women have achieved greater degrees of authority, at least in the post industrialised world, there's still an enormous distance to go in truly valuing the totality of a woman's experience.

Menstruation sometimes uses the extreme language of outrageous body symptoms, for example, gut wrenching pain, crushing fatigue or extreme vulnerability, because we have stripped it of so many of its rich stories, cultural associations and language. The powerful and magical stories of ancient cultures have been replaced by embarrassment, a vast industry in synthetic hormones to control our wayward ones, and collective sighs of relief across the country once that disturbing "time of the month" has passed.

But power will out regardless of what we think or do. A woman's power doesn't quietly slink away when it's not valued or expressed. Menstruation presents us with difficulties to remind us of its evolutionary function. At menstruation we're more ourselves, even though we may feel we're not ourselves at this time. Although not always comfortable, menstruation is our initiation into the expanded reality of ourself, of experiencing our potential power.

3. *The Gifts of the Cycle*

Moving between two worlds

The rich complexity of life is played out in the menstrual cycle: the positive and the negative, the joy and the pain, the certainty and the complete loss of meaning.

From the moment of menarche (the first period) through to the cessation of menstruation at the menopause a woman, when not pregnant, is cycling between two worlds, that of ovulation and menstruation. Ovulation is often seen as the purpose of the cycle and menstruation a necessary discomfort that women must get through to restore fertility. A hysterectomy is sometimes recommended to women who don't want to have babies, or who have already had all they want. This one sided biological view of our cycle is, I believe, part of the problem contributing to menstrual distress.

As women we need to focus on the totality of the process of which our capacity to create life is but one function. We are in fact moving between two distinct and meaningful worlds, each with their own physical, psychological and spiritual imperatives. The clues to these imperatives lie in each woman's individual experience.

At the beginning of my menstrual health workshop I ask women to give me words that describe their experience of themselves in both their ovulatory and menstrual phases. These are some of the words that tumble out for the ovulatory time:

social, sensual, confident, assertive, normal, powerful, joyful, graceful, enthusiastic, sexy, passive, efficient, productive, intelligent, unselfish, harmonious, supportive, balanced, in charge, compassionate, happy, energetic, clear, strong, focused, healthy, logical.

Most of the women see their ovulatory phase as the Good Time of the month. They feel a sense of order and equilibrium to their lives. There's accomplishment and energy, a feeling of ease with others.

Archetypically, at ovulation a woman embodies the role of The Mother, her breasts full with milk, nurturing the world — woman as carer, as peace maker. She also often feels a sense of focus, being logical (no messy emotions) and clear thinking (rather than dreamy), doing and producing, and being in control, highly prized qualities that are usually considered "masculine". In the ovulatory world a woman's head is above water. She's out in the world, and she's going somewhere.

The premenstruum, on the other hand, threatens and disturbs. The sun disappears behind clouds. Worse still the world seems to wobble off its axle. Here are some of words that women throw up for me on this territory:

alone, bloated, fat (the Michelin Man), fucked, powerless, totally overwhelmed, out of control, unattractive, clumsy, vulnerable, deep, fear, sensitive, resentful, isolation, dreamy, introspective, sad, foggy, intuitive, psychic, caustic, stagnate, raw, vicious, atomic rage, exhausted, unfocused, uncertain, separation, depressed, suicidal, self loathing/critic attack, lost, stuck, driven, irritable, wanting to hide, the evil twin, Jekyll and Hyde, ugly.

Not a pretty sight! This is the flip side of ovulation, the underbelly of life. It's as if all that's dark and dangerous has come up to grab her like a monster from the deep. She has suddenly lost the way. Lost control of feelings and a sense of meaning. She's underwater now and, worse still, swimming in murky, shark infested waters with little protection. Sometimes there's a feeling of power mixed in. But often this is an out of control power, a power that she seems to inflict on others if she hasn't already turned it on herself through self criticism, depression or suicidal feelings.

The world is now an irritant, her breasts have dried up and she has nothing to offer. If her identity is closely tied to being the giver this can be confusing, and emotionally painful when that's all she's acknowledged for.

At this time she's also full of feeling, much of it inexplicable and somehow not all hers. Small pockets of light appear in the bleakness — intuition, powerful sexuality, and big dreams — but they're usually missed in the mess of everything else.

The act of bleeding can be transformative for many women. Even those who suffer pain sometimes sense the pleasure and power it brings. Women speak of:

relief, letting go, stillness, peace, bliss, ecstasy, grounded, authoritative, dreamy, tired, spaced out.

Lara Owen, author of *Her Blood is Gold* and *Honouring Menstruation: A Time of Self Renewal*, has written that the first two days of bleeding are generally about letting go, sloughing off the tensions and concerns of the past month. We are of course literally shedding the lining of the womb and it's a great metaphor for a psychological shedding. A kind of dying for which there's nothing to be done but surrender. As we empty out, a space is created for new life to emerge: our own and of course the body's very real capacity to create life. This is a particularly acute time for "seeing" our lives and to get clear directions on what we need to attend to. It's an ideal opportunity, through ritual, to realign with what we really want to achieve (Owen, 1998).

An enormous relief after the unpredictability of the premenstruum, bleeding is still a place of ill ease for some. Menstruation needs stillness — a quality in short supply in our post industrialised, fast paced existence. Stillness can be unnerving because it's unfamiliar, it leaves us open to feelings, many of which we may be unconsciously trying to keep at bay through activity. Such self attention can be unsettling if we're not used to handling our feeling side. So sadly a woman may ignore her inner promptings to detach from the world for a while and follow the slower rhythm of her menstruating body. Unless of course she has pain and must stop out of necessity.

The feelingful nature of the menstrual phase is, I believe, a great positive. Feelings are our life blood and infuse all our actions with meaning. Without them we might as well be machines. The problem is not that menstruation exposes us to deeper feeling, but rather a culture that doesn't know how to live with this complexity. Boxed in to very narrow definitions of ourselves, we imagine we can have happiness without its counterpart, despair. What we fail to realise is that the psychological muscle that enables us to travel through the land of aching despair is the same muscle that allows us to feel great joy.

That a woman should travel through such contradictory experiences in her cycle is testimony to the length and breadth of her humanness. She doesn't need drugs to suppress the more dangerous and unpleasant aspects to return her to "normal", by which of course we mean the one sided state of ovulation. Rather she needs guidance in how to read, "hold" and value herself, and to act on her self knowledge. In the underworld of each period, a woman goes mining for more of her nature. She needs training in the language of inner life just as much as she needs training in how to manage the material aspects of living.

Simply having strong feelings may be healing in and of itself. Dr Andrew Weill, a Harvard trained physician, encourages people who are sick to cultivate passion. Whether the emotion felt is positive or negative seems not to matter; rather it's the intensity of the feeling that gives it power to affect body function. He believes that apathy, more than negative feelings, are the major emotional obstacle to spontaneous healing (Weill, 1990).

The psychological vulnerability that happens premenstrually may be a saving grace for women — it acts as a release valve for built up tensions. Sometimes the simple release of feeling is all the remedy we need. Modern drugs, with their emphasis on suppression of menstrual problems could actually be making things worse for women because they deprive us of this natural release valve.

The emotional messiness of menstruation is the antidote to too much order and predictability. It brings colour, makes us tender. It stops us from being an endless "doing machine" reminding us of our inner life and of the softer, more subtle qualities of life. It brings us down to earth, strongly connecting us with our bodies through the flowing of the blood, leading us to the earth. It takes cold logic and warms it with dreams, dreaminess and feeling. Menstruation metaphorically fills us out (a little too literally sometimes!). Menstruation itself is a kind of medicine (Slayton, 1990).

The nature of cycles

Cyclicity rules all our lives whether female or male. There are bodily cycles that spread out over an entire day (circadian), some longer than a day (infradian) and some occurring many times a day (ultradian). Going against natural body rhythms can create stress. Anyone who has worked night shifts knows how hard this is on the body over a long period of time. Jet lag is a result of your body clock literally turned upside down. And insomnia can foul up a good day without any trouble!

Imagine a doctor telling you to ignore your circadian rhythm. Ignore the natural inclination to sleep at night, just keep going until you drop. Not only would it be difficult to order society, it would be madness for your well being. But in essence that's what's happening to women when we're told to ignore the rhythm of the menstrual cycle.

Dr Ernest Rossi, an expert in the field of chronobiology (the timing and cyclicity of biological events), found an ultradian cycle of 90–120 minutes, during which there is a 20 minute drop in alertness and energy, where if you could follow your tendency you would drift off into dreaminess. During the day we're cycling through what chronobiologists call a basic rest-activity cycle (BRAC). Apparently an overwhelming number of the mind-body systems run on this same 90–120 minute ultradian rhythm of peak activity, followed by restorative troughs. All our mind-body systems of regulation, including the nervous, immune and endocrine systems, operate according to the 90 minute BRAC. Even the brain follows this rhythm, shifting from left brain to right brain dominance every 90 minutes. In recent years, molecular biologists have shown that the cell divides, transcribes its genes and reproduces its DNA according to a 90–120 minute cycle. So the ultradian rhythm operates at the deepest level of our biological being, influencing how we think and behave — we truly are time-creatures.

This suggests that we need to take regular 20 minute breaks throughout the day to maintain wellbeing and optimum functioning. The 20 minute break is a time to rejuvenate, incubate ideas and allow for some right brain creativity. Rather than it being "a waste of time", it's a window of opportunity.

Consistently ignoring body rhythms leads to stress and potential illness. This stress develops in four stages, according to Rossi, the final being when the body completely rebels and sickness occurs.

Stage one is signaled when you start to lose concentration, yawn, sigh, stretch, procrastinate, start forgetting things, and feel edgy or irritable. Is this starting to sound familiar to you PMS sufferers? At stage two you're high on stress related hormones, such as adrenaline, which will give an energy surge. If this becomes habitual addictions can kick in ... that PMS compulsion for consuming The Forbidden Foods! At stage three, what Rossi calls "the malfunction junction", we start to become accident prone, make bad decisions, spelling mistakes and fail to remember things quickly or well. At the same time we become increasingly impatient (Leviton, 1995). Rossi might as well be talking about PMS!

So, what if there were a BRAC going on in the menstrual cycle with ovulation as the doing part and menstruation that moment when you notice you want to drift off for a while? What if menstruation were a window of opportunity in which bodies could renew and psyches have space to incubate a few more brilliant ideas to action in the next activity (ovulatory) phase? What mind-body systems run on this monthly rhythm? And what if your failure to honour this is contributing to dis-ease?

Going against body rhythms is bad for your health. Any

aspect of yourself you choose to repress or ignore will one day call for attention, more often that not in a most unwelcome way. If you're comfortable with your changing nature and can easily follow its imperatives, not unlike Rossi's description of following the ultradian rhythm, you'll experience far less tension and flak leading up to and during menstruation.

4. *The Liminal Space*

Liminal spaces are windows of opportunity, a way of liberating our thinking, a place of dreaming, a time for magic, a place to garner soul food and guidance for our life. A place to collect ourselves. It's where we step out of the world, out of our mundane life, into a kind of in between territory. No longer confined by the material world, it's a place where we can travel into the farthest reaches of our selves and the universe.

When a woman moves from one part of her cycle to another she's crossing thresholds: transitional moments she must pass through as she moves from one phase of the cycle to another. Some of these transitions will feel slight, a momentary dip in feeling or rise in energy, sometimes a pain as ovulation occurs. For other women the post ovulation phase can feel intense, not unlike what many experience coming into menstruation itself — the premenstrual angst.

Both the premenstruum, when we're trying to negotiate the transition from ovulation to menstruation, and menstruation itself are liminal states. While menstruation is a place of arrival, it's also the time between, neither pregnant nor yet fertile again (Owen, 1993).

I've heard few women complain of trouble coming into ovulation as they do with moving into menstruation. This may be because ovulation is the valued state. We're comfortable with its language, unlike menstruation for which we are ill equipped. A woman often thinks she's stupid or clumsy at the premenstruum because she's dreamier, less clear in her thinking, and behaves in apparently illogical ways. She's not less intelligent — her intelligence is simply operating in a different way. She may feel less focused because she's so much more open. Women multi-channel at this time, the way mothers do all the time, operating on many different levels all at once. All women, as we're all potential mothers, have the capacity to do this! It's simply that at menstruation this talent gets amplified.

But there's more to this transition than a momentary tension. There's a "space between worlds", however brief, where the individual is neither one thing nor the other. I believe it's this liminal space that causes us the most flak.

Imagine divesting yourself of your roles for a moment. Who would you be, what would you do without the definition of those roles? It would be like suddenly being naked, feeling exposed, unsettled. The "disturbance" we experience leading up to and at menstruation could be just this. That moment of letting go of something before anything else has arrived to replace it. Momentarily we're faced with nothing. This is the nature of transitional states. When we understand this we recognise our unsettled and awkward feelings in the premenstruum as a sign that we're changing, rather than that we're flawed. We can then accommodate ourselves to allow for these changes so that we're not distressed by them.

When we let go of our roles we become exposed, permeable to the "unseen". Like a sponge we may literally soak things up. The line between the conscious and unconscious, and between ourselves and others, becomes more transparent. We can no longer repress, or avoid, the things we normally repress. It's as though the guards have gone off duty and now all sorts of interesting, provocative and unsavoury characters get to roam through the building of ourselves — especially those characters that were kept safely under lock and key down in the dungeon! Yes, all those perverse, angry, unhappy, socially unacceptable and inept sides of ourselves get liberated! Thank goodness our bodies don't let us forget the fullness of who we are. Cycles are an amazing gift.

That tender moment between sleeping and waking when dream images are melding with thoughts of the day ahead and the uninvited and unintended sneak through, is an example of liminal space. We can experience pleasant inspirations or solutions to difficult problems. A friend of mine has some of his most creative ideas at that time. Another friend uses it as an inner oracle to receive guidance for her life. But unexpressed fears and anxieties can also rattle us. It's a vulnerable moment when our guard is down and the unconscious, in both its glory and danger, can slip through.

The immune system, our physical boundary, which is more vulnerable premenstrually, appears to mirror the thinning of psychological boundaries. I've encountered a number of women who get flu symptoms before they bleed as well as sometimes before ovulation. Women with chronic health problems, such as allergies and inflammatory conditions often find their symptoms increase at these times.

Research by Dr Elizabeth Hardie at Swinburne University of Technology suggests that PMS is not linked to the menstrual cycle but to depression or irritability arising from social or health problems. In response to this the British press came up with headlines like "Premenstrual Tension is 'all in the mind'". In other words it doesn't exist! This interpretation was demoralising for women who do feel incapacitated at this time. Their suffering is real.

While I agree that PMS is connected with a woman's overall wellbeing and ongoing health problems, I believe there is still a connection with menstruation. What some people call PMS I would call an amplification of their ongoing social or health issues. The menstrual cycle isn't **causing** the problem it's **revealing** it through increased psychological and physical sensitivity. Menstrual problems, whether unpredictable moods, pain, fatigue, endometriosis or fibroids, are signaling some **overall** health difficulty.

Our ability to handle the energies that emerge in the limenal space, whether we think them "good" or "bad", is a mark of our strength. Our vulnerability isn't a weakness — it's merely an opening. Although sometimes disturbing feelings surface, our enhanced sensitivity allows us access to new ideas, visions and transcendent states.

5. *The Journey Begins*

Menstruation is a natural high, an altered state of consciousness. Intuition, psychic skills and dreaming are more developed. Who needs drugs and alcohol, when you've got menstruation to take you off?

Menstrual wildness is untrained power, a moment of alignment with our deepest selves and with something much bigger than we are. Don't be ashamed of it. Regard it as something that you're not yet skilled in the use of. Your years of menstruation are your very own self development program into the nature of that power and how to use it. Each period you're being initiated into yourself and into more expansive states of reality. Your task is to be willing to travel into the labyrinths of your self, to hold that alignment, that self knowledge, as you go out into the world.

Each month as the premenstruum comes around, you'll be reminded of what you didn't attend to or what wishes to be known in you. If you consistently hold back some frustration, you'll find yourself angry. If you gave too much to others and didn't attend to your own creative endeavours you may feel empty and irritated. Menstruation is teaching you to honour your cyclical nature.

Discovering the power of menstruation is an evolving process, each month you'll hone your skill at it. The more you know and tend to yourself, and the more you act on that knowledge, the less you'll suffer premenstrually and at menstruation.

You can begin your journey by imagining that at menstruation you're an exquisitely tuned creature. Imagine that in the premenstruum you're testing your wings to become this exquisitely tuned being.

If you want to increase your power, it's mandatory to travel into the depths of yourself, to be willing to surrender and risk feeling emptiness and darkness. You must then take that knowledge and practise your power in the world. However messy (and it is messy), with time and awareness you'll become more skilled. This is the process of initiation. And eventually at menopause you will, as they say in the Native American tradition, become your power.

Letting go

For Clare menstruation is "an unnerving time because I feel so vulnerable and uncertain. I feel taken over by something else, I am not myself. On the first day I always need to go to bed for one hour as a way to deal with it." She also suffers from deep cramps that are eased by sleep.

Planning to do a rebirthing workshop, Clare realised that it was to take place on the first day of her period (when she feels most exposed). Her immediate reaction was panic, she would not be able to take care of her needs, she would not be in control. Recognising that because of her increased sensitivity it would be a particularly provocative experience, she took time to talk herself through her fear — she had to trust she would find the support she craved at that time. Clare got more than she anticipated — for the first time, no pain — as well as the authority to say what she really needed. "I wonder if I didn't need to have the pain because I was supported in working with deep emotional states ... my wilfulness might be why I have the pain and why I don't know myself at menstruation."

Clare's fear had kept her from an excellent remedy. Apart from the cultural messages about not "giving in" to menstruation, which are enough to stop any woman slowing down, Clare is a single parent and self employed.

The altered state of enhanced awareness she was able to enter into in the rebirthing experience, had come after much inner work. So perhaps she was ready to handle this deep emotional state without being overwhelmed by it. Her fear of letting go could have been a wise voice in her psyche warning her not to be casual about what she was exploring. It held her back until such time as she was ready to engage with the charge.

Journey into power

Forthright and willing to explore, Penny had attended an endometriosis support group. She was motivated by severe health problems, including endometriosis and polycystic ovaries. Not someone to sit around, she signed up for my one day workshop without hesitation and even offered to help me set up on the day. She also informs her various doctors, including gynaecologists, about other strategies she's pursuing to relieve her symptoms.

As fearless and outspoken as Penny is, she hates, and even sometimes feels faint, at the sight of her blood. She wears tampons to minimise her connection with it. To open women to their own intuition on what might be healing for their bodies, at the beginning of my workshops I do a simple meditation and guided visualisation. Woman are often very surprised at what comes through. Penny simply saw the colour red. She admitted she was fascinated by the colour, has dreams of it and wants strong red clothing but shies away from it. Too strong. This woman is strong, but, like many of us, a neophyte in how to really ride her strength without wearing herself out.

Penny's endometriosis could be alerting her to her power and to the danger she's in if she does not come to terms with the way she uses her power and passion. Although she's only in her early 30s, I can feel the "old knowing" rocking in her, and healing her symptoms will be a training ground in how to tap this wisdom. Her loathing of her blood speaks volumes to me about her fear of this knowing. Penny agrees with me and feels through her healing process she's learning about herself.

Listening to Yourself

"IF MEN FLEE THE FEMALE, WE WILL SURVIVE, BUT IF
WOMEN THEMSELVES TREAT FEMALENESS AS A DISEASE
WE ARE LOST INDEED."

Germaine Greer

1. *Sensitivity*

Menstruation's sensitivity is a wonderful opening to the world of feeling and spirit. If you can travel through this opening with greater acceptance, you will experience over time an illumination and knowingness that will suffuse the whole of your life.

All menstrual problems are linked to sensitivity. During the transition times in your cycle, you may feel more exposed, more sensitive. In particular, those parts of yourself or ideas that you normally hold back come to the surface. If you're not being attentive, this exposure can make you feel anxious, inadequate and emotionally fragile. Your immune system is more sensitive premenstrually and you may also find yourself more vulnerable around others who may label your reactions as premenstrual mood swings.

But if you feel exposed and "seen through" at menstruation then you also have the capacity to see through facades into the depths of an issue. It's as if at menstruation your being can't tolerate denial and untruths. This reminds me of the story The Emperor's New Clothes. The emperor, through vanity, is deluded into believing he's wearing the most exquisite clothes when in fact he's wearing nothing. He is surrounded by fawning courtiers who only tell him what he wants to know. It takes the innocence of a child to penetrate the charade and shout out "The emperor has no clothes" as the emperor parades through the streets displaying his new "outfit". Like this child, your soul, through the language of your symptoms, may be seeing through the charade of the unsustainable and intolerable aspects of life.

While your vulnerability might feel like a terrible weakness, the weakest system is in fact the one that has no give in it, no vulnerability, therefore no movement and change. Without that give you would become hardened, entrenched and less able to respond. It's your flesh-and-blood feeling nature that makes you human. Your feelings are a form of knowing that can't be accessed directly by the logical mind.

For some women the feeling of exposure is a rawness so intense that they want to hide. Rather than condemning yourself for not being able to cut the mustard in the "real" world, recognise that your need to hide is the coded language your body uses to get you away for a while. It's a message that there's something else you need to tune into requiring solitude, silence and your gift of exquisite sensitivity. Don't worry if you have no idea what it is you need to tune into. When you give it time and space, this other world will come unbidden.

Premenstrual sensitivity, which often manifests as crankiness, could be nothing more than a desire to be left alone. It's not necessarily that you dislike your partner, children, or job — these elements of your life on the whole may be pretty good. But sometimes you simply need to open the front door and walk off into the sunset for no other reason than you just need to do it. It doesn't mean you're leaving forever (as your loved ones might fear) when you withdraw your attention. It doesn't mean that you're ready to quit your job. It simply means for 20 minutes, half a day or a day, you simply have to do something different. It's not always rest, although for most people rest is usually very necessary. It's simply to be, or to breathe in a different rhythm. A small shift may be all you need, but if you consistently ignore the small promptings they will become massively big ones.

What I really, really want

In answer to my question: "If you could follow your natural inclinations leading into and during menstruation, without fear of judgment from others, what would you do? What is it you most want and need at that time?" Sandra expressed a desire to head off to a South Pacific island to luxuriate in warmth, sea, sand and beauty. Sadly the state of her bank balance precluded this as a viable option! But fortunately she did not need to take her inner guidance quite so literally. What lay at the heart of it was a desire to completely drop her bundle, rest, and to experience more pleasure and beauty. Looked at in this light her desire became much more manageable and affordable.

When asked the same question, Connie simply wanted to return home to Mum. As a wife and mother herself, and also in the paid workforce, I'm not surprised she needed some mothering herself. I can't think of a better remedy for many menstrual woes than letting ourselves receive care or, more importantly, not having to attend to others!

By doing what they needed to do, these women were able to be free from suffering — great preventive medicine!

Tears also have an alarming tendency to flow more easily in the premenstrual time. What can I say? Go ahead and cry! Cry for apparently no reason. Yes, it's a sign of your rawness. Tears can release tension, tenderise you and water new growth. Cry knowing that you're exercising your feeling life, coming to a sweeter and more open place inside yourself.

By welcoming the tears, you welcome the deep feeling nature of the Feminine. Your tears are for loss of Her, as you cry your tenderness and openness call her back. By crying freely you're also opening the way for men to feel their equally strong tender feelings with less shame.

For those women who are extremely responsive, and there are some who even faint, it may be that they are sensitives. A sensitive is someone who has the capacity to pick up greater subtlety and to see beyond the material form of things. They might be able to sense the future, pick up what other people are not expressing and be more telepathic. This is a capacity to read non-ordinary reality.

Fainting could be an amplified version of a need to get away and into another reality. Melissa had an enormously stressful job and each month on cue at menstruation she'd faint. Her co-workers and boyfriend were all for her getting medical advice, certainly a wise thing to do; however, in her case she sensed deep in herself that the fainting was stress related. Sure enough once she had left her job, the fainting stopped.

I have also met a few women who faint, or experience dizziness, at menstruation who as young girls had psychic experiences which were not understood. As a result they repressed that side of themselves. Once they started to recognise their psychic abilities, the fainting stopped. Amy whose story you can read in Restoring Imagination, was a great fainter. When she acknowledged her psychic skills and creativity through art, her fainting stopped.

Witchy wise women

Witches were wise women, healers, with a talent for seeing into the mystery of things. Rosemary and Elena are two women I know who experience, in their different ways, the difficult side of being able to read non-ordinary reality. At one time they might have been called witches, or at least women with the potential to be witches.

Rosemary is an extraordinarily sensitive woman and vivid dreamer. Occasionally in her dreams she has premonitions of future events. She suffers from endometriosis and each month has to escape under her bed covers particularly just before the bleeding begins. At that moment she can't cope with anyone looking too directly at her and generally experiences the world as a psychic invasion which she is literally trying to ward off.

In her early twenties a boyfriend's father had warned him that Rosemary was a witch — he had seen women like her from Southern Italy before and they were all witches! Thinking he was quite mad Rosemary told her boyfriend not to pay attention. We laugh over this story now because maybe there was some truth in it. Sadly the father perceived her particular talents as dangerous and possibly evil and believed she should be shunned.

Elena can't stand her husband even looking at her just before she bleeds...she yells at him to look away.   During one of my workshops, I noticed throughout the day how Elena would come up with very penetrating observations. She spoke with an authority that made us all sit up and listen. I believe she was very unaware of her particular wise woman talent. Over time I thought that perhaps her inability to cope with being seen may have reflected her inability to recognise her talent for being a sensitive, for having a unique sight, which became amplified in the premenstruum and experienced by her as a terrible exposure.

2.   *Dreams and Dreaminess*

A time to wander, rather than be purposeful and driven, the premenstruum and menstruation are also a time of vivid dreams, dreaminess, vagueness and general contrariness. It's a time to give logic a rest and surf the outer realms of your psyche through your dreams, dreaminess and intuition. This is all part of the attention shift that menstruation demands.

Although logical thought may waver during this time, your intelligence is strengthened; you are making better connections between your thinking and feeling sides. Your spelling skills, for instance, might marginally take a downturn but in their place you may cook up some great creative ideas, have strong intuitions, see current problems from a wholly new angle and consequently find solutions. Going against that dreamy state may create disorientation, confusion and even headaches. So don't bother trying to balance the account books at this time if you don't want to. Instead start to recognise menstruation as the creative asset it is.

Dreaming is healing. Dreams provide access to our unconscious. Native Americans regarded menstruation as a time for having Big Dreams. These are dreams that carry greater meaning and significance than usual. In a classic study on recurring dream images, the psychoanalyst Dr Therese Benedek, working with an endocrinologist, could determine where her patients were in their cycle by looking at the content of their dreams (Shuttle and Redgrove, 1986)

In his book *The Biology of Dreaming* Ernest Hartmann comments on the similarity between PMS and dream deprivation. He found that premenstrual symptoms are worse when women don't get enough sleep and improve when they are allowed to sleep more that usual. Two women in Hartmann's study described their premenstrual tension as how they felt after a sleepless night. So more sleep could be a treatment for PMS!

According to Hartmann, REM dreaming sleep increases towards the end of the cycle, around days 25 to 30. He suggests that the changes of the menstrual cycle produce an increased need for REM sleep late in the cycle — if this increased need for dreaming sleep is missed it can show up as premenstrual tension in the daytime (Hartmann 1967 in Shuttle and Redgrove, 1986).

A tendency to dreaminess can be a clue that bleeding is close. The pattern of the dreams you have while asleep will also give clues to ovulation and menstruation. We can never have enough signs for these and you're less likely to be caught unawares!

Accommodate the dreaminess. Slow down and allow your curiosity to extend your vision of the world. Dreaminess softens the boundaries between our inner life and the outer world, opening us to surprising discoveries.

Record your dreams for the whole cycle — if you are very busy simply make a note of the significant features in the dream. The act of recording will make them more meaningful, and as in the Benedek research you may start to tune into a pattern of recurring characteristics that will indicate where you are in your cycle. Picking up these signals is another way of deepening and enjoying your experience of your inner life connected to the cycles of your body.

If you work in an occupation where dreaminess presents a real problem, such as when the public's safety depends on your ability to be focused, it's important that you're aware of your dreamy tendencies. This alone will ease tension. If at all possible, take frequent short breaks, even just a walk around the work space. Make sure to get plenty of rest and drink water through the day while on the job. Because of the electro magnetic radiation from computer terminals, you may find yourself becoming more vague and even confused. I explore this further in Part 6 on the environment.

Focusing on demand

The first day of her period and a statistics exam became a recipe for failure for Avechi. "I was sitting in the exam and there was this big wall in front of me — I couldn't see through it." Menstruation was certainly her enemy that day! The wonderful, dreamy fluid state of bleeding seemed to work against the kind of focus she needed for this exam.

But if you're ready for it, menstruation doesn't have to work against you. Janice, who's story first appears in Restoring Imagination, had a counselling session with me just before one of her political science exams, also on the first day of her bleeding. Aware of her needs and fears she had about the exam, she used the therapy session to support her tender dreamy state and connect with the inner strength of menstruation. She went into the exam feeling calm and centred, found she enjoyed the whole experience and got a well earned distinction.

Dreams are a wonderful source of guidance — nowhere is this more amplified than around menstruation. And dreaminess in general is a great space to ruminate on ideas and problems for which you are seeking some resolution. In the way we might "sleep on" a problem, I recommend women "bleed on" a problem. If it's a decision about something in their life, I recommend they "cycle on" it. That is they allow themselves the whole of one cycle to come to a resolution. The combination of the act of dreaming, waiting and observing life allows something powerful to arise unforced from within.

Wouldn't it be marvelous when next you reported PMS symptoms to your doctor, she or he reached for their prescription pad and scrawled on it: more sleep and more dreaming! So stay snug under the bed covers and dream on!

Angels and thugs

I had a dream in which a woman is murdered. She is a strong, independent woman, successful in the world. She has been yearning for a relationship with a particular man but looking from the outside into his house she sees a child's pushchair. Although empty, the pushchair suggests he has a relationship with another woman, with whom he has a child. The woman's hopes are dashed and she finds herself in dark alleys associating with dangerous company, violent men possibly involved in sexual perversion, who become her murderers. Other people in the man's house are not interested in this woman's fate. Their interest is with the woman with the child, whom they regard as the acceptable woman. The murdered woman is an embarrassment — in their eyes she had lost control, a deeply shameful act. She has fallen from grace.

My dreams have always guided me through my menstrual healing. The dangerous men have been a theme of my premenstrual dreams. I woke from this particular one feeling troubled. It had been a restless night and I felt fragile, as though I might get sick. Puzzling over the dream I suddenly remembered I was on day 21 of my cycle. Could it be that the empty pushchair was speaking to me of the passing of my fertile time, my chance of conceiving passed for this month? The dream spoke of danger, loss of control, dark underworld figures and the sense of being the outsider, a failure. I can't help feeling this is a reflection of our culture's view of the fertile woman as the acceptable, valued woman and the non-fertile woman as irrelevant and dangerous.

3.   *Anger, Bitchiness and General Provocativeness*

Anger is a fabulous energy not to be wasted. The more this provocative force is repressed in us the more she will not be reasoned with and the more destructive she will become. Of course I'm not suggesting by any stretch of the imagination that menstrual disturbances give you license to abuse or hurt anyone, yourself included. They categorically don't. But in the case of this reactive "don't-stand-in-my-path" force you have a potentially amazing ally for achieving things.

What if our angry outbursts and reactive, bitchy, "look-at-me-in-the-wrong-way-and-I'll-eat-you-alive" moods during the premenstruum were completely valid and full of juicy, potent information that was restoring some balance to our life? And that rather than apologising and banishing this provocative force to the wastelands, we welcome it in?

Often lurking in the shadows of our reactivity to the world is a discomfort with who we are and what we're doing. Sometimes we're cranky with the world because we're cranky with ourselves. Premenstrual anger can be a sign that we need to simply withdraw from others for a while, a need for solitude. Our anger gives us clues about what's really going on in our lives.

Your anger may be a signal that you have not been standing up for yourself enough or that you're out of sync with what's really important and inspiring for you. For example, you consistently ignore small irritations with your partner in the interests of maintaining harmony, and you wonder why you become a reactive monster premenstrually. Your reactivity is saying: deal with those irritations more regularly.

Extreme anger might indicate an injustice in your past, or present, which is difficult to face. For example you have experienced some trauma in your childhood that you've tried to ignore or forget. If this is the case I would urge you to seek support from a therapist to unravel the injustice and to find a more empowering way to articulate that rage. In the long term, you'll need a form of therapy that allows for healing of the original wound.

Dangerous freaky territory

Menstruation for Teri is an insane time of pain and rage. A " freaky" time, a powerful time. Before attending my workshop she had already instinctively put rituals in place to mark this time. She would leave a tampon out to signal to her partner that the "dragons had arrived" and she would play her favourite song Difficult Women by Renee Geyer. "All these radical changes each month — I don't want this — it's magnificent and its too much. The pain kind of affirms the phase I'm going through, makes me pay attention." Teri is walking a knife edge in this dangerous territory called her magnificent power. Energies are on the loose. She knows the importance of these energies, but doesn't yet understand how to ride them with more ease.

She was on the Pill continuously for 6 years until the age of 24 for contraceptive purposes. Throughout the second half of her twenties she did not remember having period problems so we must ponder at the age of 40 how much the suppression of her cycle with synthetic hormones has contributed to this extreme backlash from her body.

Teri's job as a paediatric nurse involves night shifts, another complication affecting her body rhythms. An aspect of her work that enrages her is the male doctors persisting in calling the female nurses "girls", while the male nurses seem to avoid being called boys. She feels demeaned and enraged by this, particularly premenstrually. The rest of the month she uses humour to get her through it. I believe her anger is justified and it is important that she doesn't dismiss it.

At 26 years old she started to suffer from temporal-lobe epilepsy for which she takes medication. Although the medication is necessary for her, Teri and I both suspect it could be making her menstrual problems worse. She will have to work around this one. Temporal-lobe epilepsy can be associated with strong transcendent states as is menstruation (Borysenko, 1996). There is no doubt in Teri's mind that she is a woman who senses much. Premenstrually she feels she's fighting something off, fighting to remain "out there" and "up there".

Because of her particular type of epilepsy, Teri may already have a strong tendency to altered states akin to what can happen at menstruation. Menstruation may be amplifying her experience even more. Perhaps her challenge is not to fight the force trying to come through at menstruation, but rather to let go into the energies moving her.

If anger is persistently there to meet you as you come into menstruation, I do urge you to consider some kind of self enquiry, which includes recognising the wider environment in which you live. It's important to see the bigger picture and understand your anger in context. Your feelings may not all be personal — there's a lot of suffering, injustice and intolerance in the world worthy of being angry about. Sometimes activism, rather than therapy, is the best antidote to these feelings.

Rather than condemning your anger, get this wonderful, provocative power on your side — before she creates mayhem! Doing this is the interesting challenge! Enjoying her punch and wickedness in the privacy of your own mind is a good start. Psycho drama and roleplay are safe ways to experience her as a physical reality in all her outrageous glory. Finding assertive female role models, building confidence in yourself in general and learning to stand up for yourself more in however small a way, will minimise the destructiveness of this force.

To cope with your rage in the moment without hurting others I recommend removing yourself from the situation as soon as possible and privately letting off steam. Say all the things to a cushion or chair, or even to your God/dess, that you would love to say. Let it rip! Do strong physical activity and feel the charge of the rage through your body. I've often kept a few old, chipped plates or cups on hand to smash. So satisfying, especially if you walk away leaving the bits scattered on the ground for a while! But a word of warning — do it outside or where there is enough space and no one around. Old phone books are great for tearing into when you feel you want to tear into someone. Once you've got rid of the charge of the rage you'll have a renewed clarity and the ability to articulate genuine grievances.

Although it may sound contradictory, if you're normally quick to lose your temper, it's a useful discipline to be able to hold your feelings of rage. This doesn't mean suppressing your grievance. It simply means not exploding all over the place. Ironically, exploding can also be a way of avoiding.

When you feel the anger rise in you, hold the charge of that anger inside. Feel and observe what opens to you internally as you allow the charge to forge new pathways inside rather than simply dissipate into the world. It may also help to remove yourself from the negative situation. Although I find it a challenging discipline, it can be illuminating, often allowing me to take the other person's perspective more easily.

Always remember you're having to wrestle with a cultural atmosphere that says it's not OK for women to be big, bold, brassy and loud while for men it's acceptable. Such behaviour in men would usually be called being assertive whereas women are criticised for being "aggressive". As American hip hop artist Missy Misdemeanor Elliott put it "When a guy acts in a certain manner, it's healthy aggression, but when a female acts in the same way she's called a bitch. All it really means is a female knowing what she wants" (The Good Weekend, 31 July 1999). Or as one very hard working mother said, "It's when we pull everyone into line!"

When we experience this charged angry state we're clarifying our boundaries and saying "Enough is enough".

Losing it, using it

Kylie felt bad about herself. She had completely lost the plot with her neighbour. Her anger went far beyond the immediate incident and became a character assassination of this person. Fortunately her neighbour could give as good as she got — they had had a "stand-up-and-slug-it-out verbal fight". Kylie was in her premenstruum.

She generally finds it difficult to assert herself. And guess what, rattiness and reactiveness come pouring out like flood water breaking the dam just before she bleeds. A generous hearted exuberant women with a terrific sense of humour, I sense in her a regal spirit with which, I suspect, she is unacquainted as yet. I can't help imagining that it's this regal spirit, a force with enormous authority, which gets totally pissed off with Kylie's failure to assert herself sufficiently and which comes through, all guns firing, in that limenal premenstrual gap!

Her therapy work with me is a slow, gentle, gutsy, funny journey to help her appreciate her bigness of character. I imagine, with time, she won't so much lose it premenstrually as use it to enhance her authority in the world.

4. Depression, Loss of Meaning and Self Loathing

"If we have the courage to face into the dark we may witness the slow epiphany or showing forth of the feminine" (Hall, 1980, p.19). The feminine knows the necessity of darkness for the creative process. The seed germinates in the darkness of the soil, the foetus grows in the darkness of the womb.

Because we have difficulty appreciating dark states, we can tend to feel cast adrift from ourselves and the world, disconnected from all meaning and purpose. A common experience for many women just before, and very occasionally after, bleeding. For some there may simply be a temporary collapse of spirit, a blue feeling and sense of self doubt. For others it can be an intense feeling of hopelessness. Women who suffer from clinical depression, like those who suffer chronic health problems, may also experience an amplification of their symptoms.

Depression is a turning inwards, sometimes so much so that our thread back to the world may feel completely severed. When we feel depressed we may perceive something that's too painful to know, or too overwhelming to grasp, or act on. Perhaps the knowing is more "in our bones" than in our brain so it's hard to articulate. I think at the heart of depression is a great longing to feel a deeper meaning and to experience more profound places in ourselves. Ecstasy, a quality deeply imbedded in the menstrual experience, is the other side of depression.

After an event has occurred, usually a painful one, women

will often say she "knew" or sensed what was happening all along but because the idea was painful she would push her knowingness to one side, later to be confronted by the truth. If she had been able to act on her hunches she may have felt more empowered.

Despair may also have a direct link back to a painful past trauma. This despair is one you can normally cope with but your menstrual sensitivity won't now let you. Or menstruation may be intensifying feelings of depression at not having conceived, or not being able to conceive.

Just as anger rises in you about injustice in the world, your depression could also be a response to the many despairing events happening in our times. The 20th century was after all the most brutal century on record. How can we not feel an incredible bleakness about the way we are treating each other and the planet?

Depression can sometimes be our psyche's need to escape from superficialities. I can't help speculating that the relentless "upbeat" atmosphere of urban life is enough to make anyone feel down. Not having to be continuously up and out there being seen and getting ahead can sometimes be a relief.

To sometimes feel empty and lost is a normal experience and a part of life. Of course you deserve to be joyously happy — I don't wish depression on anyone. But the more we run from such feelings the more monstrous and out of control they'll become. Because depression usually slows us down, even stops us altogether, it's the natural companion to ceaseless activity. Your down times are the doorway to exalted states — with depression as your co-traveller you will also be able to experience great joy.

Your sadness and emptiness inform the joy and plenty. To experience these exalted states you need to risk going into the parts of yourself you don't like — those dark and empty places that you catch out of the corner of your eye but usually keep at bay with such things as activity, food or television. Emptiness, loss and sadness will be there to greet you. But if you go with these feelings rather than fighting them you'll find their opposites will come to you more easily.

So, cradle yourself through the premenstrual downturn being aware that "to know" you must have moments of complete "not knowing" — a healthy dose of doubt. And remember that when the blood comes the cloud will lift. For some women there is even a dip again on about Day 5 or 6 of the cycle. Don't forget that as we move out of menstruation we enter another transitional moment into the ovulatory world.

I believe this postmenstrual "dip" could be linked with a woman's overall health. If in general she suffers from chronic fatigue symptoms, the loss of blood may overly weaken her, leaving her emotionally more vulnerable. The Chinese believe that at menstruation a woman loses chi, or essential energy, also possibly accounting for this "dip".

Life is cyclical and we humans are not exempt from that rhythm of generation and regeneration, of death and rebirth. In Western culture we're fond of the rebirth but not very good at accepting the dying or letting go. We imagine that death is always followed by more death when in fact it is "… always in the process of incubating new life, even when one's existence is cut down to the bones" (Pinkola Estes, 1992, p. 135).

Around menstruation, when you feel yourself descending into darkness and emptiness, remember this. It's better to find someone to help you learn how to go with your depth of feeling, than it is to medicate it. We have a natural ability to regenerate after such experiences and useful though medication can feel in the moment, it may be depriving you of that renewal and a life greatly enriched from the experience. I am not referring here to those of you who are being treated with medication for a chronic depressive illness that is strongly present whether you menstruate or not. If you're taking medication it's vital that you don't stop taking this medication without consulting your health practitioner.

Self loathing

A vivid feature, and perhaps even the cause, of the menstrual "down" time is a sense of self loathing. Suddenly you find yourself under the penetrating gaze of your Inner Critic. This self examination can cut deeply into your core and paralyse you. Or in turn have you lashing out at the world as a way of deflecting the internal attacks. Either way it's bleak.

This critical voice is the part of you that is condemnatory, puts you down at every turn and doesn't believe in you. It enjoys pointing out what you have failed to achieve rather than acknowledging your successes. It's a constant in most women's lives but its voice becomes even more penetrating and shrill in the premenstruum. It has a way of getting you to examine everything you think, feel and do … and, guess what, you usually come out wanting in its eyes.

Sometimes in my counselling practice, a woman will come to a session cast into the deepest pond of despair. She is but a day or two away from her bleeding, or has just ovulated. Nothing is working. After all the months of therapy she still feels she has got nowhere and is ready to give it up. Yet when I see her at the next session (yes, she's decided to come to one more) the previous despair is forgotten. It might as well never have existed. Although she may feel better it can be a risky position. The more she disowns her despair the more it will rise up and bite her each time the period comes. But those women who continue to attend to themselves will find the dips ease over time.

Why is the inner critical voice able to wreak such havoc at menstruation? It's because your defences are down — that vulnerability at work again. I believe to cope with this you need to become more comfortable with self examination. It's good to be called to account for what you're doing. Are you doing what you really want, are you being true to yourself, are you valuing who you are? Remember, a little doubt is very healthy.

Your criticism, whether of self or of others, will often hold a kernel of truth. You need to attend to this truth. So, after you have peeled yourself off the ground or picked up the recipient of your criticism, don't wholly back track on what you have said. It's often the way the criticism is delivered that's problematic and needs apologising for, not all of the content of what was said.

Loathsome though that inner critical voice can be, it's challenging you to stand up for yourself, and if you really find you can't justify a particular aspect of your life, treat your critic's penetrating observations as a catalyst for getting you to change what is truly not working. Recognise your premenstrual self examination as a being-called-to-account moment. While it's challenging, with awareness and time, it will make you stronger.

If you're particularly tough on yourself, which can also be reflected in being judgmental of others, I would recommend you see a psychotherapist. She or he can be an ally, helping you stand up to this challenging voice. Facing your inner demons can be a delicate and slow process.

If you can learn to ride the cyclical ups and downs with greater acceptance you'll develop an incredibly useful and resilient psychological muscle that will prepare you for any major life challenge. To go Up and Out into the world, you need to be able to go In and Down. Menstruation is one of those useful In and Down moments.

Facing the inner critic

Jackie came to me for therapy because she felt bleak and devoid of meaning. When she didn't have to work she would often take herself to bed not wanting to connect with anyone. Nowhere was this need more acute than in the premenstruum.

She had almost no faith in herself, and our work together was a slow recovery — to learn to stand up to her inner critic, to credit herself with the things she had achieved which were numerous but which she often dismissed. Getting out of the work she came to hate, and finally finding a relationship in which she felt loved, were also vital in helping her to find some lightness and meaning in her life.

As her life improved, her premenstrual downturn also improved. She still retreats just before she bleeds. When she makes that OK for herself, rather than fighting her need for solitude, her depression lessens. She becomes OK **in** herself.

5.   Addictive Tendencies and Loss of Control

Who among us has not felt that compulsion to eat sweet and rich food, particularly chocolate? Often as we approach our bleeding, we no longer feel our own person. Food cravings loom larger than life. We also tolerate alcohol less easily which means we get drunk quicker on less. This sense of loss of control can be so strong for some women they feel they are being driven by something else. In a culture that prizes control and order, this feeling of "losing it" can be acute and difficult to tolerate.

Menstruation is its own natural high. There's a shimmering clarity available for a woman who can allow herself to enter menstruation as an altered state of consciousness. When I talk about addictive tendencies I am really talking about losing touch with ordinary consciousness — like being flipped into another state of being.

An experience of this is vividly described by Natalie Angier in her wonderful book *Woman, An Intimate Geography*. "One of my most beautiful memories of college is of a day when my period was due but hadn't yet arrived. I was sitting in my living room, studying, and I felt an unaccountable surge of joy. I looked up from my book and was dazzled by the air. It was so clear, so purely transparent, that objects in the room were sharply etched and proud against it, and yet it was as though I could see the air for the first time. It had become visible to me, molecule for molecule as though I had taken the perfect drug, the one that has yet to be invented; call it Liberitium or Creativil." (Angier, 1999 p. 98)

I was not aware of the full strength of menstruation until I was in my forties, although I can remember being filled with enormous surges of feeling that I often did not know what to do with. I suspect that while we may be gifted with moments of this shimmering clarity and joy in the early years of menstruation, it is only with time and self knowledge that we are able to access this state with regularity and increasingly heightened glory. One of the advantages of getting older!

Loss of control premenstrually is an abiding theme amongst the women at my workshops. It can range from binge eating through to extreme emotional reactivity. One women felt so out of control with her anger that she seriously felt a danger to the community. I believe that any woman who has addictive problems with food, (bulimia, anorexia, binge eating), alcohol, sex or drugs, may find the liminal state of menstruation will exacerbate her addiction.

Perhaps we're drawn to food to try and blot out the rawness of feeling, the sense of exposure. If we don't understand the highly sensitive state of menstruation we may fall into patterns of self loathing or anxiousness. Reaching for some comfort food, for example, is a way to dampen the vulnerability that leaves us open to yukky feelings.

Your biochemistry can also greatly affect your moods and cravings. Low blood sugar, serotonin and beta-endorphin levels can result in many of the characteristics associated with PMS such as tiredness, confusion, difficulty concentrating and remembering, irritability and getting angry unexpectedly (low blood sugar); depressed, scattered, suicidal, reactive, craving sweets (low serotonin); low self esteem, tearful, reactive, overwhelmed by other's pain, depressed and hopeless, craving sugar (low level of beta-endorphin) (DesMaisons, 1999).

If you live on a diet high in refined carbohydrates (e.g. white bread, cakes, sugar, alcohol), foods high in hydrogenated fats, and few vegetables you will be contributing to this biochemical imbalance and exacerbating your hormonal changes. Do you crave sugar premenstrually? Blood sugar levels are famous for performing great acrobatic diving feats just before bleeding — they can drop resulting in sudden craving for something sweet. Beta-endorphin levels are also at their lowest in women just before menstruation. This can also create cravings for sugar. Reaching for some chocolate may provide sugar. But rather than balancing the levels, it will send them skyrocketing. To get caught in this cycle is destructive and will push you further from the goal of greater emotional and physical ease. Following the diet I recommend in this book will put you on the path to biochemical balance and your mood swings will be reduced.

Cravings for sugar or junk food can also be an indication of mineral deficiency. Mineral deficiency is inevitable if your diet is poor and it's worth having a hair analysis to find out your mineral status.

At menstruation a woman loses iron with her blood. This loss of iron has a protective function for the heart, but too much iron loss weakens. I know women who suddenly have an enormous craving for a great slab of steak before bleeding whereas for the rest of the month they rarely think of eating meat. We need fuel for the bleed. Perhaps in part your craving to eat may be Nature's way of making sure there are reserves of fuel in the body. As long as it's the right fuel of course!

It's hard to imagine how this "out of controlness" can in any way be useful when all it does is make us put on weight or look foolish, for example from drinking too much, or having an emotional outburst.

Perhaps our cravings are also a metaphor for our need to refuel in general. To "take in" after "giving out" to the world. Recognising your very human need for nourishment at all levels over time will restore greater balance and ease psychically and physically.

Eating sweetness

Could your sugar craving be something as simple as wanting more sweetness in your life? Sandra recounted how she goes out to buy a bag of jelly beans — it has to be jelly beans — then hurriedly and secretly eats them all. She categorically does not want to share them. This was a woman who for most of her life had put her energy into bringing up her children. They were now leaving the nest, and much as she loved them she wanted them to go. I cannot help feeling that, as a mother, not much would have been sacred to her.

It truly is a psychological necessity to have moments of total self indulgence, or at the very least to acknowledge the need. Unfortunately jelly beans are full of sugar and synthetic colouring agents which would only exacerbate her symptoms. She needs to find another way to nourish her soul.

Menstruation is an opening to a numinous space. Our addictive tendencies could simply be the shadow side of our inability to recognise this wonderful altered state. They may be mirroring the ecstasy, bliss, or paler versions of this that are seeking us at menstruation. So rather than try to rebottle the wild genie start to ride with her. Don't condemn yourself for your altered state of consciousness — become curious about it.

6. *The Language of Physical Symptoms*

The voice of illness

When she was diagnosed with fibroids, Anahit's uterus was the size of a four and half month pregnant women. Already on a good diet, she suspected stress was the culprit. Although she liked her job, it was extremely demanding with a less than supportive environment. She was also completing a Masters degree, as well as coping with her mother's life threatening illness.

After much reflection and inner work Anahit chose to have an operation to remove her fibroids. She found a surgeon who was very supportive of her way of coming to terms with the course of action, and his sensitivity gave her confidence in his skills to do the operation well.

Although she decided to have the fibroids removed, she also chose to explore them imaginatively rather than running from their presence. Beginning by doing drawings, she heard a very grumpy voice reminding her of the women in her family, her grandmother and mother, complaining about their difficult lives: accumulated resentments against men, hard work and the struggle to make a new life in another country. Working with both a psychotherapist and an acupuncturist she allowed herself to physically feel the fibroids as well as gain a mental impression of them. As she went deeper into the experience imaginatively they came to symbolise a strong still character in her. A character that takes a lot to stir it, that has a lot of life experience. It accepts what comes and goes. It's about eldership.

I believe that the strength and resilience that comes from

enduring hardship is the other side to the sufferings of the women in her family. What looked like grumpiness revealed itself as a wise deep strength. This is possibly Anahit's inheritance from these women.

The underlying message for Anahit was that she needed to love her fibroids more. This is another way of loving herself. She's also learnt she needs to love the baby part in her, the sweet cries, and to grieve the fact that she may not be able to have a child. This is helping her connect to tenderness, and in her words, a deep connection to the Divine. "I have to drop my agenda and be with what is. It's living with uncertainty."

Through her fibroids Anahit is coming to love her womanhood, her strength, the power of tenderness and vulnerability, and the courage to risk going for what she deeply wants. She has recognised that she has a strong, still, wise voice inside herself which she must show in the world more confidently.

If you're suffering physically you may feel angry with your body for letting you down. You may feel despair, or perhaps simply a low grade resentment, a kind of ongoing cold war. It's normal to feel this way and acknowledging these feelings may be necessary before you can move on. The process of reimagination, which above all means discovering and experiencing meaning, may help you to accept your suffering.

When I talk about physical symptoms I include all premenstrual discomforts such as bloating, weight gain, constipation, diarrhoea, nausea, headaches, even pain. This also includes conditions such as endometriosis, fibroids, cysts, polycystic ovaries, PID (pelvic inflammatory disease) amenorrhoea (absence of a period) and irregular cycles.

Symptoms are an important wake up call to attend to your health more assiduously. They are guiding you to knowledge of yourself and overall health — not some arbitrary whim of a willful God sent to taunt you.

Your personal experience of the physical symptoms is your guide. Any body disturbance is a device attracting you to yourself and urging you to pay more attention to the situations you're in. Taking notice of your physical symptoms can shake you up and shift you out of entrenched positions. You can use your symptoms, the way Anahit describes in her story, to bring forth more of your talents and to acknowledge yearnings and hurts that you might otherwise ride over.

As you start to reimagine your suffering, your warring feelings could continue to resurface. Again this is normal. You need to keep feeling them in order to find the life beyond them. Imagine that the physical symptoms are pulling you into your body, particularly the lower part of your body. Think of them as encouraging you to become more embodied, to be connected and comfortable within the body you have.

Being in touch with your body means you'll become more in touch with who you are. The requirements of physical symptoms have a way of distracting you from activity and leaving you exposed to what is truly happening inside you. Initially this can be unsettling if you have uncomfortable feelings such as low grade depression, an unrequited or unacknowledged longing, or a self loathing that you usually keep at bay through activity and engagement with the world.

So start paying attention to your symptoms. Stop and give in to the experience. For example, instead of stuffing down lots of painkillers so you can "keep going", give up the "keep going" agenda and travel instead with where the pain leads you. Coming off pain killers will be easier to do if you follow some of the many practical suggestions I make in later chapters. Your understanding of yourself will be both revealed and changed by the simple act of listening to your feelings and your body. Even when you do take painkillers, don't force yourself to do inappropriate things for a body that's suffering.

A client who had no knowledge of my menstrual work, happened to comment in passing one day how, when she chose not to take pain killers for her period pain one month and instead lie down to rest it out, she had incredible revelations about her childhood and family difficulties.

Your detailed observations of your precise experience will also provide vital clues for your health practitioner. With any symptoms you experience, note down things like where the pain or discomfort is, the type of pain and the pattern of it.

Personal trauma, particularly sexual abuse, may be connected with physical menstrual problems. While it's still sensible to pursue very practical remedies for the physical suffering, a tender self inquiry with the support of a sensitive psychotherapist may also be very necessary.

As you feel both physically and imaginatively into the experience of your fibroid or that cyst on your ovaries or the lack of a period altogether, you might begin to sense things about yourself. You might have hunches or intuitions. You're tapping into an inner guiding knowledge, like Anahit who began to hear the complaining voices of the women in her family which later she recognised as a resilience and sturdy inner strength that she needed to trust more. You might become acutely aware of how you block your creativity. The pain of your endometriosis could be alerting you to a gutsy, maybe angry voice that is circling now in your uterus. All that bloating and weight gain is perhaps a signal to pick up your bigness of character! Have fun with your imagination, if you can. What's important is that there's meaning in your personal experience of your symptoms, not that the fibroid, endometriosis or other problem mean something specific. You're the only person who can unfold that meaning.

The power of pain

Severe pain each month has proved an enormously grounding experience for Anna. She chooses not to take painkillers wherever possible but rather to really feel the pain. "I let myself go into the pain, I try talking to it, feeling it — there's an enormous repressed anger and strength in that pain. The pain is unbelievable — so extreme it's like being burnt at the stake."

Even though she has a very sharp, intelligent mind Anna sometimes feels quite light-weight. She has an enormous sensitivity, even a feyness, which is certainly not valued in the academic culture where she studied and now teaches. Consequently she feels easily judged and can be self critical.

The pain literally pulls Anna into a deeper strength within herself, a "primal sense of being" which she really likes. She has learned to ride the pain and, through it, believe in herself more fiercely. She becomes more gutsy and determined to face those forces that she normally feels threatened by. "I feel my pain is a cry against the one sided atmosphere of academia. I feel all the ways that women are crucified and that amazing hushing up of who I was. I've known it since a child, rebelled against it while inevitably being drawn in." The pain is like a great unnumbing process.

She also actively uses her menstrual cycle as the inner guidance system it is. When dealing with difficult life decisions she will give herself the menstrual "month" to dream and reflect on the issue. The bleeding is the crunch moment when she listens for her deep knowing on what direction to take. I have observed her rise to the challenge of the authority that arises from her being at those times. I'm inspired by that.

With time, her inner knowledge and authority will infuse the whole of her life. Perhaps the pain will recede as she does this, or perhaps she'll still need to attend to a strict diet and pursue other alternative remedies.

The womb cannot be ignored. It's as though you have to think and move from deep within your pelvis. In traditional Japanese martial arts the most powerful movement is one that comes from the koshi or pelvic region. Learn to use your physical disturbance as mind/body awareness training to ground you in the present. It does take courage to do this. It helps if those around you understand what you're doing so that, in your personal environment at least, you don't have a negative undertow pulling you back from inner knowledge and healing.

In time you'll become clearer about your boundaries, about what you can and can't take on, what are and what aren't your responsibilities. Suddenly what was fuzzy will come into sharper focus as you begin to recover knowledge. Knowledge that's critical for healing your body and revivifying your spirit.

Using the Power of Menstruation

"THE VALUE WE PLACE ON MENSTRUATION HAS A DIRECT
CORRELATION WITH THE VALUE WE PLACE ON
OURSELVES AS WOMEN."

Lara Owen

1. *Honouring Your Soul*

As women we're blessed in having the menstrual cycle. Without needing to think about it we're reminded naturally to attend to ourselves. Traditionally women are seen as the givers of nourishment, the mothers. But we also need to be mothered, to become takers and receivers, as well as givers. Menstruation simply alerts us to this. Menstruation reminds us of what's important in our lives, and what we need to pay attention to. Of course, these are things that we need to continually attend to, not just at menstruation. But it all gets highlighted at that time.

To heal and maintain wellbeing we need to do some things just for ourselves and no one else. We need to feel as though our life is meaningful and going somewhere. We need nourishment that permeates all the layers of our being. And the more lasting remedies are those that help us explore the meaning in the disturbance of menstruation, that guide us in restoring a sense of the sacred to our beautiful bodies, and build our sense of self worth. If we don't nourish our souls and our bodies at menstruation, our needs will leave their calling cards.

Many women, I find, are edgy about too much self attention. It smacks of selfishness — even self obsession. I'm sure you can be that at times. But your personal needs don't disappear just because you're not attending to them — they'll strike back in a coded language that is far more disruptive.

Good diet is revolutionary for resolving health problems. But it's not a substitute for the food you need to give your soul. Soul food is the things that inspire you, make you want to get out of bed in the morning. It's about following your passions. It's the celebration of imagination. Soul food can also come in quite inconsequential forms: the thrill when a storm breaks, waking up to a pure blue sky, the warmth of your cat as she snuggles up to you, silence, a piece of music, the smell of your child … Soul is also about experiencing meaning. It's about feeling the sacred, alive and pulsating in all your mundane, everyday activities and objects..

The clues to what feed your soul come from those things that lift your heart, get you curious. The things you find yourself coming back to again and again. This has nothing to do with what your logic tells you is "right" — for that you might just conclude what's socially acceptable, sensible and, well, logical. Useful though logic is, understanding the nature of soul life is the one place where logic is way out of its depth.

I've heard many people say they feel far removed from their passion, as if they are just subsisting. Sometimes people who, on the surface, seem to have it all — a great job, partner, children, plenty of money — still experience inner emptiness because they're not in touch with their soul needs.

My mother worked part time as a cook for many years for a closed order of nuns. One of the few outsiders to be allowed in, she became extremely close to the women. She was fascinated by why they would choose such a life. The Abbess, who before she entered the convent was a student at university with, it seemed, a great future ahead of her out in the world, replied "I got the call, I was furious!" I love that! You can't argue with your deep inner imperatives — when they speak you have to act.

Because of increased sensitivity at menstruation, we're much closer to our soul voice. Our symptoms are the soul voice speaking. Forget being sensible — it's time to follow your whims and passions. So follow that voice rising up from the deep well of your being. Sometimes this voice is asking you to do something that feels very difficult and challenging. And yet you must do it.

Allowing yourself to surrender more and more to your tendencies at menstruation will naturally open the door to soul, to the rich imaginative feeling world, to the intangibles of life, to Mystery. With time you'll cultivate this depth of experience, and it will spread like a delicious atmosphere through the rest of your life.

When you open yourself to your soul life you're deepened. You can move with greater fluidity between the upside atmosphere and the underside of life, the outer and the inner, between your logical, analytical skills and your gut-knowing and intuition, your mind logic and your heart logic. Both are very necessary and when you accept both you may find you feel more connection between all things. It's as though the privileged sight you feel so acutely, and maybe crazily, at menstruation, is a talent you can begin to draw on throughout your cycle.

It's a healthy part of life to have doubts about the direction you choose. But when you attend to your soul needs, your life will start to feel pregnant with meaning. If you experience menstrual suffering, especially premenstrual despair, it could be because you're not doing what you want to be doing, have lost touch with what you want, or perhaps you don't know what you want. You may not be fulfilling your creative or soul needs.

Creativity is to do with the way you live your life not just whether you have a natural talent for the arts. Unless you're an artist such as a writer, painter, musician or inventor, you may think you aren't, or cannot, be creative because you don't have those particular talents. But your life itself is a creative act — you are the artist of the life that's unfolding for you. It's this life that is meaningful.

Attending to creativity is powerful medicine. I'm not referring specifically here to our awesome potential as a woman to create life (although having a baby is routinely prescribed by doctors for the menstrual dilemma). As humans, women and men, we are creative beings.

You may be thinking: "Yeah, but my life is unfolding in an uncomfortable and unhappy way and it all feels pretty pointless." Yes, it can feel just like that. But what if your menstrual symptoms were, in this case, part of the creating voice speaking to you of your talents? Like any challenging or painful experience your symptoms are part of the artistry of your life.

I believe there's important information in the mess you're experiencing — your task is to unfold it. Even if you don't know how on earth you'll do it, try to find this information. To begin, try looking on yourself with less hostile eyes and you may find a softening occurs. In that softening you may start to notice more — significant dreams, greater awareness, increased acceptance, sensitivities, synchronicities, intuitions, inspirations. Yes, menstruation itself can be a creative moment.

There's nothing like curiosity for discovering something in the most obscure data. It's not so much about finding the job you're meant to do but to experience yourself as meaningful.

Creative and meaningful work

Helen had a very painful menstrual history, physically and emotionally. She associated her bleeding with abandonment as her parents suddenly split up two weeks after her first period.

She struggled through her twenties in a great deal of pain. Her doctors, she felt, were disparaging — appendicitis was even suspected at one point. It took eight years to be taken seriously, and get the diagnosis of endometriosis. She had an operation to clear the endo and briefly tried the drug Danazol, but found the side effects so horrible — gastro intestinal problems like bloating, heart burn, nausea and weight gain. Worst of all, her legs would suddenly go numb. With no sense of her legs being there, she felt they could give way without warning. This sensation unnerved her and prompted her to stop taking Danazol as she felt there were no benefits from taking the drug.

When her endo symptoms returned she consulted a naturopath. For two months she had intense treatment — herbs, massage, chiropractic work and acupuncture and her pain greatly diminished.

Two years later she began to make and sell cloth menstrual pads as she was very concerned about environmental hazards associated with disposable pads and tampons. During the time that she was working on this business her pain stopped altogether! I was so surprised I had to get her to tell me this story three times to make sure I had heard it correctly! When she stopped making the pads because it was proving to be unprofitable for her, the pain returned. On reflection, Helen realised that when she was making the pads she was doing something that felt very right to her. Menstruation guides her to what feels creative and meaningful.

Many women find meaning through the arts — writing, drawing, making music and working with clay are some of the ways to explore your suffering and release feelings and frustrations. Working with these art forms can open the door to meaning. Anyone can do this, it requires no particular talent other than a willingness to just do it.

Put yourself into a quiet space where there will be no interruptions. Take a little time to tune into your experience of your symptoms, drift internally with whatever thoughts, sensations or images come to you, and then pick up the medium you choose to work with and let the internal experiences flow out without censoring it. This doesn't have to be a work of art!

Write without hesitating. If you do find yourself hesitating, repeat the last word or sentence, but just keep going. Forget about spelling, punctuation and grammar. Just keep going. The more you write the easier it will become. It's very important not to think too much, just write. And you may also sometimes enjoy being slower and more reflective as you write.

I have written to my journal as a friend: Dear Journal ... and I have poured out all my despair and frustration. Sometimes I have written to a wise part of myself. I call her the wise woman: Dear Wise Woman ... and I have told her about hopelessness and feelings of impossibility. After I have written to her I put down my pen, sit quietly for a moment, then pick the pen up again and write: Dear Alexandra. She is now replying to me. At the end of the piece I sign off as the Wise Woman. I have stunned myself with the words that have flowed from the end of my pen. Wisdom, useful guidance, genuine inspiration and comfort. I have read back over these letters months later and they still move me.

When drawing, notice what colours you are drawn to in your paint or crayon box. Let the images form as you put the colour to the paper. Or perhaps you have very clear images of the "thing" inside you, that insane pain, or hard lump. Draw it! The act of drawing, or even working with clay, as with writing, will lead you to a place you didn't know about before you began.

Making sounds or music can work in exactly the same way as the drawing and writing, engaging you in a visceral experience of your symptoms, bypassing the logical mind and accessing a deeper place of knowledge. They provide opportunities to channel feelings that might transform into something unexpected, moving and powerful.

If you feel drawn to the arts and would like to explore this form of therapy more deeply, you could consider working with a professional art, music or dance therapist. You don't have to have any particular talent, or training in art, music or movement, to benefit from these therapies.

2.   A Sacred Time of Rest

Menstruation is a time of renewal for our whole being. Lara Owen calls it the Sabbath of Women (Owen, 1991). The practice of Sabbath was originally connected with the ancient Babylonian Sabbatu which comes from Sabat, meaning heart-rest. In Babylon it was a day of rest, occurring once a month at full moon. This was when the goddess Ishtar, the goddess of the moon, was said to be menstruating. Travel, work, and eating cooked food were prohibited for both men and women on this day. These distant days of rest, linked to the moon and menstruation, were the origin of the modern Jewish Sabbath and Christian Sunday (Owen, 1998). I can't resist Tom Robbins' tongue in cheek response, "So nowadays hard-minded men with hard muscles and hard hats are relieved from their jobs on Sundays because of an archetypal psychological response to menstruation!" (Robbins, 1980, p. 22)

Implied in the word Sabbath is the notion of menstruation as sacred time. I like the idea that our time is sacred. The Yurok Indian woman believed menstruation was not something to be wasted on mundane living, but to be used to explore the meaning of your life. Our premenstrual out-of-sortness is a gentle (in some cases not so gentle!) reminder of the need to attend to matters other than the everyday. The difficulties we experience as our blood flows is a deepening of this experience. This makes menstruation a particularly potent time for rituals, prayer and meditation.

Menstruation restores knowledge of the sacred and majestic within ourselves. Stepping into menstruation is like stepping into a sanctified place such as a church, cathedral, mosque, temple or special place in nature. Cherish and hold in your memory the sense of presence, the silence and the majesty of those places as you are filled by something beyond yourself. Remember this as you bleed. At the heart of this sacred moment is the act of surrender. It begins with something as simple as an attitude change, although to fully feel the depth of this place you must stop what you're doing and be completely still.

I believe the need to slow down a little around menstruation is normal. It's our body prompting us to rest for a while rather than waiting for an illness to force us to stop. Obviously, if you experience extreme or, for you, abnormal fatigue you've been pushing your boundaries. Chronic menstrual fatigue must be taken very seriously as a warning that your body is run down and that you're in serious need of care.

In our speedy times we equate fast pace with efficiency and productivity, with excitement and therefore with a life worth living. Slowness is vastly underrated. But speed is wearing, it cauterises feelings, does not allow for depth of connection and the savouring of life. Constantly moving in the fast lane means being constantly hyped. Apart from becoming addictive, this is also deeply wearing for the body and soul.

Slowness is restorative to all aspects of our being. It restores the fullness of our senses and feelings, allows for reflection and simply being, for response rather than reaction. You may be surprised to discover that you're no less efficient and productive simply because you're more aware and centred. In fact, you are likely to be more effective and efficient.

So, be radical: take a stand for slowness! And remember that men need to slow down just as much as women — it's just that women have a built in monthly reminder to change pace and go inwards for awhile. Never let your need for this be regarded as a weakness.

Dropping out

Gloria used to say to her family as her bleeding began that she had a migraine and needed to lie down. But she didn't have a headache, she never did — she just wanted to drop out of the world for a few hours. To her way of thinking menstruation wasn't a good enough reason to do this — after all we're not supposed to be changed by menstruation. We're supposed to be like men (the same all the time) and able to ride over things. As if that were a good thing and as if men could actually do that too! Gloria didn't know why she wanted to lie down and disengage from her husband and children, she just did. She felt bad for wanting to do this accompanied by a very real fear that she might be judged. Rest is often seen as a weakness, and wanting time alone is regarded as a bit weird. In fact isolating oneself is often seen as a sign of a psychological problem. So to bypass these cultural codes, Gloria dreamt up a migraine headache. At the end of my menstrual health workshop I was delighted to hear that she had decided to dispense with the headache myth, replacing it with a sense of pride of her period as her Sabbath. She was simply going to tell her family that she wanted some time alone.

Rest is unbeatable. I call it a little known ancient remedy that costs nothing and is highly effective! If women could rest more at menstruation I swear menstrual problems would be halved overnight. Time and again women react when I say this. They say they can't afford to stop, feeling that if they do they will not "make it" to positions of power in their work and in the community. The life of our uteruses has frequently been used as an excuse to keep women out of high office or any office or workplace for that matter. I've said it before and will keep saying it — stopping, hanging out and doing nothing, are necessities for all human beings.

We must stop perpetuating the myth that feelings, slowness, and wanting to be quiet and alone, are symptoms of weakness. In reality, the weakest person is one who is unable to handle non activity and quietness. None of us can afford not to stop. And now you are about to become the radical one who spearheads this change! Just in case you're not quite up to this warrior role yet, keep quiet about your need for rest to others, but be honest with yourself.

Although some women are very supportive of the need to retreat, I have sometimes found that women who don't suffer at menstruation can be the most intolerant. As women we could do each other an enormous service by supporting each other with our menstrual needs.

So if you want to bury your head in the sand for a few days or stay under the bed covers, go and do it. I'm well aware that while you literally may not be able to close shop for three days, you can for an evening or for half an hour or so. Even as you go about your business there's a way of letting go internally. A woman once described to me how she coped with a very demanding job while menstruating. She imagined herself deep within a cave. On the surface she acted "business as usual" but inside she was relishing the snugness and stillness of her cave. I had the sense this helped her work with far more self composure and authority. Imagination is powerful!

Simply move at the pace of your menstruating body — you'll discover this is much slower than your normal pace. When you move more slowly you'll notice so much more. Not only that, you'll be in touch with the intrinsic power of menstruation which will fill you with a greater sense of sovereignty.

As far as possible, I do seriously encourage you to find ways to fully rest. This is an absolute necessity if you have difficult symptoms, and if you don't, it's preventative medicine for maintaining your good health.

When you fully rest, your soul and spirit are nourished and your body is repaired. You allow another kind of wisdom to come through which you can only access in stillness and silence. This doesn't mean flopping in front of the television. It means allowing yourself a completely empty space to contemplate, meditate, or just drift and dream. It means being rudder-less for a while and allowing yourself to be carried by your internal tides and currents. Allow yourself to welcome what comes to you: creative ideas, solutions to difficult problems, visions, powerful dreams, bliss ... and healing.

Menstruation reminds you of your time. Exteriors dim and your interior becomes lighter. Make yourself unavailable. Don't go the extra mile. Allow others to pick up the slack — you'll find they're perfectly capable of doing so. And even if perchance they're not — well, let the world be a little less perfect. Trust that the world won't come to an end if you're not fully on the job. Burn your list of things to do. Allow yourself to be surprised at the serendipitous things that can occur when you let go.

3. *Creating Ritual*

Ritual is powerful. It's our way of honouring something, marking a moment as significant. We use it to take us through difficult times of passage, such as the death of someone, or for celebration of beautiful moments, such as the birth of a baby or the coming together of two people in marriage. In our modern, fast paced world, we have also lost some rituals — particularly those that mark rites of passage such as puberty and menopause.

Ritual marks a territory around something. It says this is sacred space and sacred time, whether it's to celebrate or to grieve. We need rituals to help pass through limenal moments, whether those moments are painful ones such as the loss of a job or the end of a marriage, as well as to celebrate the joyous transitions.

Often transitions are double edged, such as when a baby is born. It's an amazing moment and yet extremes of feeling can coexist. Some women slide into postnatal depression. Inevitably there is grief for the land we're leaving, despite the joy of the new state we're choosing. It's as though we must honour the spirits of both the old and new worlds and failure to do so will lead to disturbance. It's not unlike the thirteenth fairy, the one that wasn't invited, turning up to "curse" the new born baby of the king and queen in Sleeping Beauty.

Ritual, like power, will seek expression whether we do it consciously or not. We all have ritualised elements of our lives — often referred to as habits. Perhaps a habit is a ritual acted out unconsciously. Habits are comforting because they're familiar and act as a container to hold our lives. But habits can also be destructive too because of their unconscious, and sometimes uncontrollable, nature — and perhaps because they are no longer connected with any sense of the sacred.

A ritual that acknowledges the menstrual cycle with its light and shade, the purposefulness and emptiness, is a way to lift the curse of the uninvited — all those messy uncontrollable symptoms — and turn them into something useful and meaningful. It's a way to honour and amplify the power of menstruation.

The ritual of charting your cycle symbolises a special attention to yourself and your extraordinary body. There is something both powerful and intimate in knowing what's happening in our body at any given moment. I feel it myself, and women speak of it to me, especially those women who have recently come off the Pill and are rediscovering their cyclical nature.

You can make your chart as simple or as elaborate as you want it to be — moving from recording physical changes such as mucous and temperature, changes to the cervix and breast sensitivity, through to emotions, intuitions and dreams. These changes will all give clues as to where you are in your cycle at any given moment which is vital for contraceptive and conception purposes. For example, as you approach ovulation the mucous will become more profuse and clearer like raw egg white, your temperature will take a sudden dip and then rise indicating ovulation has occurred. Some women have quite distinct pain alternating each month between the ovaries, which can be a sign that ovulation is occurring. Francesca Naish's book *Natural Fertility*, has excellent instructions about charting for conception and contraception.

Keeping a journal and writing down what you experience through the bleeding itself is also valuable. The more aware you are and the more information you record, the richer your experience will be over time. The discipline of observation will make you more perceptive. Knowing where you are in your cycle means you'll be prepared for any difficulties and disturbances.

Alas, for some women their very problem is irregularity, which makes planning for menstruation just about impossible. Nonetheless, charting the irregular period may in itself reveal patterns and over time this attention could generate regularity.

Another ritual to mark menstruation is to wear a special item of clothing or piece of jewelry. A Sydney company, Full Bloom, which makes the most wonderfully comfortable bras, have designed a pair of underpants from leopard skin print with a red gusset for women to celebrate their bleeding.

Wearing cloth menstrual pads, rather than disposable pads or tampons, can be a ritual act. If the great selling point of the disposable pads and tampons is the fact that you won't notice your blood, then cloth pads will surely focus your attention on menstruation like no other thing! But in the nicest possible way, as you will discover when you wear them! In the words of one young woman: "Menstruation can be a bit of a bummer but with the (cloth) pads it's all right!" Washing the cloth pads, instead of being a burden, can also become a ritual — a ritual of closure, that will mark the transition from the menstrual to the ovulatory world.

Giving yourself permission to do absolutely nothing at your bleeding is a ritual. This is particularly powerful if you are generally a "driven" person. Be tender and sweet, take the phone off the hook, switch off the mobile for 24 hours (I mean it!) and surrender. Feel all the cells of your body release tension, tiredness, toxins. Let your being empty of all the stuff of the past month … everything. Cry, ache, dream, and dream some more. Bliss out.

Simple acts of grace

Janice takes to her bath at menstruation for a long soak followed by a self massage using a special blend of aromatherapy oils.

Kirrilee will use the special charge and heightened awareness she feels at menstruation to create a ritual to bring about something she wishes to manifest in her life. Placing a large sheet of paper on the floor, she uses words and art to pour out "all the emotional stuff going on in my life". When she finishes she goes the other way and writes about what she wants in her life, gives herself compliments and draws a positive image. Sometimes, if it's a warm day, she'll take off all her clothes and allow herself the pleasure of feeling the blood flow while she's writing and drawing.

Teri has an altar which she uses as a place of comfort when her premenstrual suffering is bad "I sit in front of my altar and talk to Crazy Woman. It's like a meditation, a prayer time. I talk through what I'm really feeling and therefore I can connect with what is causing the problem".

If you're a woman who is trying to conceive, or would like to have a child but are not in a situation to do so, then the sight of the blood is a moment of real grief. Far from menstruation bringing ecstatic feelings and visions it may be filled with tears and despair. Ritual can be helpful at such a time. You could try any of the previous suggestions but instead it would be your grief that you are marking. It's important not to run from your grief each month. Instead, talk to your body, cradle your yearning and bless yourself with some simple treat.

Celebrating puberty

A passionate advocate for menstruation, Amrita Hobbs has developed puberty rituals to support young women in their transition from girlhood to womanhood. Many young girls, because of their embarrassment of menstruation, absolutely don't want any recognition, acknowledgement or, worse still, celebration of their first period. However, I heartily encourage parents to find some positive way to mark the transition. Although she may not thank you at the time (although don't be surprised if she does!), that positive regard will have lodged in the sinews of her being and quietly feed her a message of her OK-ness.

It's never too late to have a puberty ritual! I was present at one of Amrita's ritual gatherings which was recorded by the Australian Broadcasting Corporation in which the age range spanned 14 to 40. Such rituals can help those of us at any age who experience incompleteness from our transition to womanhood.

If you find yourself fighting my ideas about ritual, feeling the silliness or the impossibility in them, try to follow the suggestions anyway. Even as you don't believe in them — go on and try them anyway. Try them grudgingly, but keep going. Each period just take one small step …

4. Tapping into the Power of Love

Discovering love

Puberty for Deva was sheer hell. Her period did not come, her breasts failed to develop. She had such bad acne on her face and around her eyes she could hardly see. And she shot up in height 10cm in one year due to too much testosterone.

Her father, an emotionally abusive man with extremely high expectations of his daughters, would laugh at her and call her a freak. By not intervening, Deva's mother failed to protect her. And if it had not been for the insistence of a friend's mother, Deva might not have got medical advice.

At age 17, on seeing the doctor, Deva felt for the first time her problem acknowledged. He was furious with Deva's parents for not bringing her in sooner. She was placed on the Pill, got a period and her acne cleared up. Because she had polycystic ovaries, the doctor advised her to stay on the Pill for the rest of her life. She took the Pill over the next eight years, with the occasional break when her period would stop.

Suffering from depression, at the age of 19 Deva discovered Transcendental Meditation which she became very committed to and which kept her sane. In her early twenties she completed a university degree and took off for India where she found Buddhism. While she was in India she had a strong instinctual feeling that she wanted her period to be generated without drugs.

Initially, Deva consulted a Tibetan medicine practitioner and then later met a woman who offered to give her weekly massages for two to three months. Through the tenderness of this touch, Deva felt that she was experiencing love for the very first time. Six months after stopping the Pill her period came. She was ecstatic! She is now in her 30s and has a period every month. Her blood tests reveal that her hormones are balanced although she still has some cysts around the ovaries. Deva's mother had ovarian cancer and Deva has recently been advised that if she doesn't stay on the Pill she too runs the risk of cancer. Although she agrees with her doctor's theory, she chooses not to take the Pill and continues to work with natural medicines to maintain her wellbeing.

Deva feels that there was a connection between her menstrual problems and lack of nourishment, the ingredient most missing in her childhood. Yet it was not physical but rather emotional and spiritual nourishment that she lacked. Through healing her menstrual difficulties she was able to find this nourishment. A quiet dignity has grown from her suffering, a surety about who she is and the life she has chosen.

Love is a great remedy. It's what this book is all about: our capacity as women to love ourselves, to love our bodies, to love the power of the Feminine. Without this kindness to ourselves it's difficult to get in touch with our inner knowledge and to find the doorway to genuine power in the world.

Entering the menstruating years (menarche) is such a mixed bag for many young women. Sometimes there's a genuine excitement but soon this can be worn down by the apparent inconvenience of it all and the wall of public embarassment and silence that surrounds menstruation. For many girls there is only shame and sometimes even anger — a sense somehow her body has betrayed her. Yet, menarche could be a joyous moment, one of great pride and dignity at stepping into womanhood. Any loathing of her body at such an important moment in her evolution severs her from an inner authority.

This severance can be deeply wearing and even potentially sickness making.

How you feel about yourself will make a difference to your healing. Healthy self esteem, or self love and respect, is excellent medicine. Women with PMS often find it difficult to take a stand for their own needs. Healthy self esteem means you're able to make the practical changes necessary to improve your menstrual health. If you feel good about yourself you'll have no trouble asking for what you need in order to heal. You'll feel you deserve to be well. If you have a low self opinion you might be harder on yourself, ignoring your health needs. Self respect is good for the immune system and a vital immune system is your key to menstrual health.

In case you're starting to have a low self esteem attack just from reading this information, remember that many people have low self esteem and are fighting fit. They are blessed with strong constitutions. Your symptoms are not a signal of inadequacy.

Good self esteem means being able to take your own side. It's about being able to take and respond to criticism. It's an ability to talk to yourself in ways that are supportive when you do feel wounded and vulnerable. Good self esteem doesn't mean never having yukky feelings but rather it gives you the ability to feel the full range of your feelings. Healthy self esteem is a kind of inner flexibility that allows you to explore different points of view without feeling annihilated. It also gives you the ability to allow yourself to be supported by others.

You can build your confidence and self esteem through achieving things in the world. Small things that lead to bigger things. Make sure you acknowledge those things you have achieved, however small, rather than constantly harping on about your failures, which of course you will have as well.

Sometimes it's helpful to have an ally and that's where counselling can be useful. This is particularly helpful for women who suffer from menstrual problems or other physical difficulties. In my psychotherapy practice I've worked with a number of women with severe period pain, endometriosis or fibroids — conditions that can whittle away at even the healthiest self esteem!

When we condemn our body and messy feelings we're feeding the cultural cringe around anything to do with feelings and bodies. We're conforming to a very limited view. Women who suffer from menstrual problems often carry the loathing of all that is of the Feminine for everybody else as well, including, of course, men's dislike of their own Feminine nature. When we curse a part of ourselves, we condemn the whole.

At menstruation, you may not understand what's happening with your body, and you may feel enormously distressed. But you're not an out of control monster, even if you feel like one sometimes! There are indeed parts of you that do want to break free. Your goal is to be able to let those parts break free while maintaining your dignity and without abusing yourself or others.

Menstruation is unique to women — recognising its power may just open the door to self love. Love is the nourishment our beings most crave. There is no more potent a remedy than this and rather than wait to be loved by another, we need to seed this force in our beings and in the world. I believe that most of us, consciously or unconsciously, are convinced we will love ourselves only when we are loved by another. Loving ourselves might feel well nigh impossible. Yet, just as when we hate a part of ourselves we condemn the whole so when we love a part of ourselves, we bless the whole.

If you start to think of menstruation in a positive and loving way it will infect the way you feel about yourself. I believe this kind of thinking is contagious. It leaps from one woman to another. And the more women relish the power of menstruation, and themselves, the more men will also start to be infected by the affection! Tenderness is a great way into this self loving business. Practising tenderness with yourself at menstruation you'll find a dynamite remedy.

Talk to your body

Talking to your body is another way into this "self respect" business. When we suffer difficult and painful symptoms our body can easily feel like a hostile enemy with whom we are definitely not on speaking terms. But when you engage with it respectfully, it might respond in surprising ways. If your cycle is very irregular, try talking to your body. Ask, politely, that it start now to find its own regular pattern.

My shiatsu practitioner suggested to me once that bleeding at full moon might be more supportive for me energetically. About two weeks later, on day 19 of my cycle, I bled at full moon precisely! I was gob smacked because, impossible though my period was in those days, it was, at least, as regular as clockwork.

Recently, despite my best efforts to book a long haul international flight that was away from my menstruation, my cycle readjusted itself! I was either going to be bleeding in the final frantic days leading up to the flight or as I was about to board the plane. Either way it was going to be unwelcome. I needed it to be late and it hadn't done that in years. What else could I do but talk to my body? I simply kept telling my body that I wanted the period to start as I arrived at my destination. It did. Precisely. As I walked through the arrival gates at Heathrow after my 22 hour flight I could feel the tugging in my belly. The telltale sign that the blood was beginning to flow.

5.   *Managing Stress*

A little stress gets you going — too much of it and you start to unravel. If you lead a very stressful life, one look through this book is probably going to send your stress levels through the roof! You're already up to your eyeballs with things to do and now you've got to sort out your diet, get regular exercise, and take time out to meditate on the meaning of your life ... what a luxury when you barely have time to breathe!

But the ideas in this book are not luxuries, they are necessities. If you don't take stock now you could be in much worse strife further down the track. **Remember, the menstrual cycle is the stress sensitive system in women.** So think of menstrual symptoms as an early warning sign for your overall health.

Stress causes many physical symptoms and researchers have shown that between 80% and 90% of all illness is stress related (Pelletier, 1977 in Leyden-Rubenstein, 1998). There are many studies validating the connection between the mind and the body. In other words, what you're thinking and feeling can have consequences for your health — even short term stress can affect immune system function.

While learning relaxation techniques is a useful way to manage stress, time is the key issue. When you're stressed you don't, or feel you can't, take time for yourself. Your situation is untenable and needs to be changed — a relaxation technique won't do that for you!

Feeling under stress is also a signal that you need to stand up for yourself more. Your stress is an opportunity to take a personal stand. You've probably been saying "yes" to others too often and "no" not often enough. If it feels scary to become more assertive, it's worth joining a support group or getting counselling.

While individual women have their own personal stresses, all women are placed under stress by sexism. Sexism means valuing one sex over another. For centuries women have been in an inferior position to men, and while we have made some headway with equality, there are many continuing inadequacies and injustices. Ultimately male values still dominate in the places of power in the world. Sometimes on the surface you may find things look OK. But if you're in the company of men and you end up feeling inadequate, used or humiliated, sexism could be at work.

Sexism eats at a woman's sense of self, it implies that her fundamental nature is not OK. In particular, women are worn down by very limited images in the media of what's considered beautiful. And menstruation itself is not a topic for comfortable conversation.

Feeling continually under stress is bad news. Either you must find a way to get out of that situation, or change the situation in some way. Your situation may look impossible. But the one thing you do have some control over is how you think. Hold in your imagination how you would like to experience things. Visualise what you would like to do at menstruation. Keep holding this, wanting this. Don't worry about how you're going to achieve this — there's power simply in your imagination. The idea is like a magnet — with time it draws the means to realise what you want in all sorts of ways you had not conceived possible. Try it and you'll see!

New life, new dignity

Suffering from both endometriosis and strong premenstrual mood swings, Suzannah went through a very stressful process to salvage her marriage. Feeling betrayed by her husband's infidelities, she swung between rage and deep self doubt which came to a head in the premenstruum with strong suicidal feelings. Her period is the barometer for the stress levels in her life. After many months of attempted resolution with her husband she finally got up the courage, and her own financial means, to leave.

Within their relationship she had allowed herself to be cast as the one with the "problems", both emotional and physical — once she was "fixed" the relationship would be OK again. An unwise assumption to have of anyone at any time, but hard nonetheless for Suzannah to overcome. In the end, leaving was the only way she could comfortably recover her power and dignity.

About a week after moving out she got her period. Despite feeling exhausted from the move, all her premenstrual despair fell away and the pain was mild enough to manage without the painkillers she usually relied on. In recognising and honouring her needs, her stress, and in turn her menstrual difficulties, were significantly reduced.

6.   *Moving Energy*

Crampy pain, too much blood, fibroids, constipation or all those reactive or depressed feelings are an indication that the body's internal energy is not flowing well. It's as if the body is forming roadblocks, sending you on detours. Or like a river bursting its banks. Metaphorically, each of these symptoms speak of energy flowing in awkward and challenging ways, or deciding not to flow at all.

I've encouraged you so far to follow the movement of what you are experiencing, to go along with the ride your body is taking you on, following the curious detours and paying attention to apparent obstructions. I've urged you to stop if you feel tired, to feel into the despair rather that jolly yourself out of it, and to become more conscious of the power that manifests as cranky reactivity, instead of condeming it. This honouring will greatly relieve your symptoms.

Another very important way of working with the body energy is in a more literal sense through physical movement and body work. Exercise is hard to beat as a way of healing many of the body's woes. There's no escaping it. Exercise is one of those non negotiables in life — you just have to do it! It's necessary for all aspects of wellbeing, not just menstrual, helping to minimise life threatening illnesses such as cancer and heart disease. It keeps your body toned, mind sharp, helps ward off depression and keeps your bones healthy. The health of a woman's bones after menopause is directly connected to the exercise she did or failed to do in her teenage years.

Menstrual symptoms are like stuck energy. Exercise literally helps to keep energy flowing in your body and helps alleviate these symptoms. Primary dysmenhorrea (menstrual pain that's not associated with any disease such as endometriosis) will ease considerably, if not disappear altogether, with regular exercise. Herbalist Susan Weed in her book *The Menopausal Years, the Wise Woman Way* tells of a woman who got rid of her fibroids and cramps within three months of beginning a vigorous exercise program.

Just as humans come in all shapes and sizes, so does exercise. Some body types need a good workout while others respond equally well to the subtlety of tai chi or qi gong movement. Your guide to what kind of exercise is right for your body can come from what you naturally feel drawn to do. Find a type of exercise you can enjoy so that you feel motivated to continue and getting healthy doesn't become a joyless regime for you. This health stuff is not about punishing yourself! Although if you feel naturally drawn to being a couch potato, exercise a little doubt on this one!

Walking is great — it costs nothing and just about everyone can do it. Particularly powerful for healing are the body disciplines of yoga, tai chi and Feldenkrais. Yoga, based on Hindu religious philosophy, uses particular movements and poses with the aim of withdrawing the senses from external matters, and traditionally unites the human soul with the Universal Spirit. There are also specific exercises in yoga and tai chi for strengthening the uterus and pelvic region, and balancing the endocrine system, that, with practice, will have a direct effect on easing menstrual symptoms. Tai Chi is a series of smooth, flowing movements based on Chinese martial arts to promote balance and energy flow. Feldenkrais is another movement discipline that, as with yoga and Tai Chi, builds strength and flexibility as well as deepens awareness. It's worth telling your teacher about your health problems so they can give you specific guidance.

If you need music and rhythm to exercise, dance! Bellydancing is a wonderful celebration of the female form, its movements concentrated on the pelvic region making it an excellent form of exercise for banishing menstrual woes.

Always be careful not to overdo exercise as it can have the counter effect of weakening you. This is particularly so if you suffer from chronic fatigue. Finish exercising before you run out of energy. While moderate exercise prevents calcium loss, an excess of strenuous activity sets the stage for calcium loss at about the same rate as in postmenopausal women. It's therefore very important if you're an athlete that you follow calcium conscious practices more carefully than others (Pitchford, 1993).

Rebounding is a great alternative if you do suffer from excessive fatigue, or are just too busy to fit in trips to the gym or yoga class. The rebounder is a mini trampoline. In the privacy of your own home you can exercise. Rebounding gently exercises every cell in your body, increasing circulation and encouraging lymphatic drainage. The lymph system helps to move the toxins out of the body. Rebounding also tones the organs, including the endocrine and reproductive systems (Naish, 1993). This is perfect for women experiencing menstrual problems — the uterus and related systems get a workout in the kindest way!

Although enormously energising, if done very gently rebounding actually doesn't feel like exercising. So it's ideal for anyone who is very weak. Done before bedtime it can sometimes improve sleep.

Exercise, like relaxation techniques, will help you deal with the effects of a stressful life. It won't solve the stress but it will help you to release built up tension. If you feel extreme rage, strong exercise is a great way to burn off some of the charge. It may also make you a little more clear headed.

To get relief from your menstrual problems, you will need to exercise throughout your cycle, not just as menstruation approaches. In fact the pre-menstruum may be the time when you feel less inclined to move. While you're bleeding I encourage slowing down to just the gentlest of movements. Some yoga poses are a winner for dealing with cramping while others are not recommended while you're bleeding (check with your yoga teacher). Some pain seems to demand activity, while other pain demands being firmly tucked up in bed. Everyone is different so follow your instincts.

Know your limits

Most menstrual information and education aims to normalise menstruation, promoting the message that it's a perfectly normal, healthy process that will not hamper a woman in anyway. Very true. But in our determination to empower, particularly young women, we are sometimes less tolerant of the vulnerability menstruation brings, particularly for those with menstrual problems. Urging women and girls to do strenuous exercise, when a gentle yoga class may be more useful or even, dare I say it, A Day Off, is irresponsible. Girls and women are often taught that the solution to their period pain is not to indulge it, when I think that is very thing the pain and she needs.

Rather than imposing the mindless idea that we should keep going at all times and not give in to anything, I urge parents and teachers to listen to the clues that their daughters and students give. In particular, girls need to be taught to recognise that pain is not normal and must be attended to. They need to learn that a little tenderness and slowness may help as much as moving the body can and that sometimes a little tenderness and slowness is great anyway, suffering or no suffering.

When used wisely, exercise is a fabulous remedy. When it's a tough physical regime mindlessly imposed on your body regardless of your condition it becomes a health hazard.

As well as heading for the gym or yoga class, it may be beneficial to head for the masseuse, the chiropractor or osteopath. Body structure affects all bodily functions. If you're structurally out of whack it could be contributing to your menstrual problems and may require gentle body work with a health practitioner. Many chiropractors and osteopaths work with the body in subtle yet effective ways that involve minimal or no physical manipulation.

Period pain responds particularly well to body work. Having a massage just before your period, or on the first day of bleeding, can do much to alleviate primary dysmenorhrea. Having a gentle massage may also be perfect for your frayed premenstrual nerves: a little tender loving care if you're not able to get it from other sources. A client of mine found that her period pain, which had already eased with careful attention to diet, improved considerably after six months of weekly or two weekly Shiatsu massages. The clotting eased and the blood flowed more evenly.

Reflexology, a special form of massage done on the feet only, benefits the whole body and can be beneficial in relieving premenstrual symptoms.

Our sedentary lifestyle plugged into the ubiquitous computer, as many of us are, means that the body is cramped into limiting positions for overly extended periods of time. Sitting in chairs, especially if the seating is poorly designed, will directly affect the vitality and strength of the pelvic area and lower back.

Start to take notice of how you tense up in your lower back and belly. Learn to relax into your pelvis, find gentle movements and gentle thoughts to ease the tension. Do it as a daily, mindful exercise.

A touch of tenderness

Because of extreme pain, Rebecca, at age 22, ended up in hospital every period. When she was 15 she had been taken to hospital with suspected appendicitis which resulted in a laparoscopy and the removal of her appendix. At 18, on her first visit to a gynaecologist, she learnt that this had not been necessary and that her "appendictis" was probably her first attack of pelvic inflammatory disease (PID), diagnosed, along with endometriosis, after a second laparoscopy. At the same time she had an operation to correct a retroverted uterus and cancerous cells were found on her cervix. She took antibiotics for the PID for three years with a few breaks of several weeks in between courses. Understandably, Rebecca also suffers from frequent depressions.

In the week between the two sessions of my menstrual health workshop Rebecca had a period. She told me: "I didn't have to take pain killers, I could manage the pain." Gobsmacked, I wanted to conclude it was the power of my workshop that had done it! Perhaps there was a teeny weeny bit of truth in that as she told me, "I had never really talked about my problems — maybe talking in the group helped. I took more time to think about what was happening with the period and I went more slowly."

I questioned her further to see if she had left anything out in her story. She said that just over a week before coming to part one of the workshop she had gone to a chiropractor and had been told she had a twisted pelvis. The chiropractor had worked gently on her for an hour. Apart from attending my workshop she had made no other changes — so we can only conclude that it was this body work that made the difference, along with her greater self awareness and tenderness.

When Rebecca came to my workshop she believed she would be imprisoned in her pain for the rest of her life. Six months later she told me she had continued working with the chiropractor Rebecca gets immediate relief after each session, including one miraculous experience in which after 6 weeks of bleeding and considerable pain, both stopped by the following day.

After changing her diet, which took some time as she didn't believe it would make a difference, and giving up smoking she reported feeling "A hundred times better. I have more energy, I've lost a lot of excess weight and look healthier than I ever have. Besides that I'm much calmer and happier. I still get abdominal discomfort and some pain but it's relatively mild (although being emotionally upset often makes it worse or triggers it). The bleeding used to last for weeks and has now reduced to two days. I used to be on quite a lot of medication daily (for pain as well as a mental illness) and now I'm on none at all — I feel absolutely wonderful!"

Experiences of sexual abuse may also cut you off from awareness of problems in your pelvic area. It's essential to receive expert therapy to heal the wounds of the trauma of sexual abuse. Apart from the psychological wounding in particular to your sexuality, you may also have been physically damaged, for example the pelvis being put out of alignment.

Connecting with your body

Bella was severely sexually abused in her childhood and began her menstruating life with very bad pain. As she got older the pain eased a little and later, when she began therapy, the pain eased some more. Over a five year span she also received much osteopathic work. In her words: "My pelvis was a mess from the abuse...I think I know now not to clench up."

During a beautiful experience in a yoga class, the teacher encouraged the students to focus on their sacrums, that place at the base of the spine. Bella had her period at the time and was in pain; however, when she really concentrated on her sacrum, her pain stopped being pain and became simply intensity. As her awareness expanded she could feel the contractions of the muscles causing the pain. She kept her focus and suddenly the thoughts in her head became silent and a beautiful tingling happened in her spine: an electrical pinging in the sacrum ..." I was enveloped by silence. This is what sexual energy is, life energy, really pleasurable. I had an impression of the livingness of my bone. I was left feeling a sense of warmth, awe and pleasure and drifted off to sleep."

Sexual abuse can sever you from experiencing the beauty and pleasure of yourself and your body. In that moment Bella was able to taste bodily pleasure perhaps for the first time in her life. Such moments are pure gold that no medicine can replace.

Sexual energy is also very beneficial for menstrual difficulties — orgasm will ease period pain as it softens the whole pelvic area of the body. In fact, any therapeutic practice that leads you towards greater connection with the beauty of your being and body is worth pursuing.

Whatever form of structural work you choose, it will be beneficial for your overall wellbeing, not just your menstrual health.

Nourishing Your Body

1. The Joy of Healthy Eating

Healthy eating is critical for wellbeing. There's no substitute for it, no short cuts and no medication that can overcome the effects of a poor diet. Food also gives us enormous pleasure. And pleasure is vital for wellbeing.

Changing your diet doesn't mean you're going to give up that pleasure, it's just that the pleasures will change. With your new diet you may find yourself enjoying the sensational taste of real food, fresh minimally processed whole foods, ideally organic. You might actually like the sense of wellbeing you experience. You'll be delirious at not having period pain any more and will positively praise this way of eating from the treetops! So rather than focusing on what you're giving up, think about what you're gaining to heal your body — a vibrant healthy life.

Time and again I've seen great improvements in menstrual symptoms through changing diet. Just giving up wheat in the form of bread, pastas, cakes and biscuits, and dairy products can be transformative. Occasionally I meet women who, despite following the strictest diet, still suffer. I believe there's something even deeper calling these women. The good diet is still important but they still need to seek out the skills of a health practitioner to probe further.

Food is a highly emotive issue. What woman, at some point in her life has not thought about dieting? Guilt-free eating is probably a rarity for most of us. I'm mindful that I'm now about to give you more instructions about the do's and don'ts of food! So it's important to tread carefully and lightly.

If you're a woman with a history of anorexia, bulimia or

binge eating, paying attention to diet is probably not the place to start your menstrual healing work. If you're not already working with a psychotherapist, or don't belong to a support group, I recommend you start now. Managing a new diet might be fraught with difficulty for you and making peace with yourself and your body first will still support your menstrual health.

When you make health changes, particularly if they're radical ones for you, your body could go through what's known as a "healing crisis" — you might feel worse before you feel better. For example, fatigue and nausea might temporarily increase until your body adjusts to the new, healthier diet. Drinking plenty of water, taking gentle exercise or practising yoga can help with this. If you feel you're going through a healing crisis, go slowly with the changes, but don't stop them or you'll go back to square one.

Your weekly food bill will probably rise when you change your diet, particularly if you begin eating organic produce. Because diet, including quality food, is so important to good health, consider making savings in other areas of your life.

Changing your diet can also be disruptive to personal, work and family life. Many a time in my workshops women have resisted these health changes because they weren't willing to change their current lifestyle. They have wanted their bodies to fit in with them and not the other way around. And there's the rub because the whole essence of healing involves change. If you suffer from menstrual problems, there's something about your current way of living that isn't working for you. It may be the expectations you have with your work or how you should be as a mother, wife, partner or friend. Or it could be the personal regimes you've set for yourself that allow little time for contemplation and rest. Or perhaps you're constantly "doing" for others and not giving enough back to yourself.

I'm entirely sympathetic towards women who resist changing their lifestyle. Feeling that same resistance myself I almost became angry once with a practitioner for suggesting certain things! The change that's needed can feel completely overwhelming, particularly if your partner, family or friends don't fully understand or don't take your condition seriously. So move with caution, but never give up on your quest which is so critical for wellbeing.

Hanging in there

Katerina had been diagnosed (via laparoscopy) with extensive endometriosis only a few months before attending my workshop. Although she had had most of the endometriosis removed with laser treatment, the severe pain had returned, her periods were irregular, and she felt nauseous and tired much of the time. She had had irregular periods from the beginning, and for about ten years in her 20s was on and off the Pill. The first sign of any pain came in her late twenties, but did not become a regular occurrence until her early 30s. At the age of 30 she got pregnant by accident while using a diaphragm. She was very happy about the pregnancy but sadly her partner wasn't. He told her he wanted her to have an abortion and left the relationship. Handling the abortion on her own was a nightmare, particularly as she bled almost constantly for three months after the procedure. Katerina believes it was this enormous physical and emotional upheaval that contributed to her menstrual problems.

Coming from a medical family who had no interest in alternative medicine, listening to the dietary information in my workshop wasn't easy for her. Katerina found it hard to believe that anything like diet or acupuncture could work. At the time she was considering taking Zoladex, the drug recommended by her gynaecologist, but after listening to other women talk about their experiences with hormone drugs she decided to give natural therapies a go. Initially she was overwhelmed by the number of things she needed to attend to — when we got to the bit about giving up caffeine she rebelled: "No way am I giving up my coffee!" She did however apply herself to the bits of the diet she could cope with and also began acupuncture and Chinese herbs.

Progress was slow but she was consistent — she continued to make changes as and when she was ready for them, and stuck with the changes she did make. After eighteen months she even gave up coffee, realising how it was feeding her anxiety — because she knew it was time to stop it wasn't difficult to do so. Now, four years later, she has no pain, her cycles are regular and her energy levels are good. She recently had another laparoscopy (three and a half years after her first surgery) as she has been trying to fall pregnant. The gynaecologist was very impressed with her general and menstrual health and this time found only mild endometriosis.

Because Katerina has been dealing with chronic fatigue as well as pain, she may need to maintain a stricter health plan than most. What's important about her story is her slow pace and consistency. Some women leap in at the deep end while others start at the shallow end and slowly entertain more depth. Katerina is one such person, showing that it's no less effective if you take your time. And she's no longer skeptical of the efficacy of diet and Traditional Chinese Medicine!

A healthy digestive system

A healthy digestive system is as critical for wellbeing as good food. You can eat the most wonderful food in the world but if your body can't absorb it well you're still going to be in strife. If you're not absorbing the food well, chances are you're not effectively eliminating wastes from your body either. This means a build up of toxins which further hinders wellbeing.

My impression from years of working with women with menstrual problems, is that digestive difficulties are always present in some form or another. If you have any kind of chronic digestive disturbance such as wind, bloating, pain, chronic constipation, diarrhoea, or irregular bowel movements you may need to seek professional help along with making healthy changes in your diet. If you don't attend to these problems you'll see little improvement. I can't emphasise this enough.

If you're on the Pill, take heavy doses of painkillers each month to manage your menstrual pain, or other drugs to manage endometriosis, be aware that they put extra strain on the liver and may destroy the friendly bacteria in the gut. You need both a healthy liver and plenty of friendly bacteria in the gut for wonderful digestion. And you need wonderful digestion for wonderful health!

A healthy food system

One of my biggest health care concerns is the quality of food today. Along with water and air, food is the fundamental fuel for our bodies. Although we have a wide variety of food available this doesn't necessarily mean we're well nourished.

The quality of our food is decreasing with heavy use of pesticides, chemical fertilisers, growth hormones, antibiotics and vaccines, and genetically modified foods. Agribusiness farming denudes the soil of minerals which in turn affects the nutrient content of the food. And the confined conditions in which animals are kept and the unnatural ways they're fed to quickly increase weight, to my mind cannot create healthy food. Eating meat produced in this way is essentially consuming distress.

Processed foods contain preservatives, colourings and other additives, and may also now contain genetically engineered ingredients. The integrity of the food is affected even further by adding synthetic ingredients which may be toxic to the body and, in the long term, cause possible damage to the DNA. Denatured foods that may contain toxic solvents, used to extract fat, include those labelled: fat-free, diet, decaffeinated, defatted, lite, imitation or polyunsaturated. I suggest you avoid these foods altogether.

While scientists in favour of genetically modified (GM) foods say they have research to indicate the food's safety, this research is not sufficiently independent or fully peer reviewed and can't take long term effects into account — only time can tell us that. Because the research hasn't been conducted on humans, we don't yet know the effects on our health.

Genetic engineering allows genes to be transferred across species' boundaries from any living organism into any other. Nature also doesn't confine herself to the arbitrary boundaries we put around fields to separate crops. So there's nothing to stop these genetically modified organisms escaping into the environment and creating mutant genes, upsetting the ecology and contaminating food that isn't modified.

Diversity of food control is also critical. The control of seed supply, currently in the hands of only a few corporations, doesn't bode well.

Because of inadequate labeling of GM foods, the only way to make sure you're eating quality food is to buy organic or biodynamic or grow your own. When buying organic you'll also be doing an important service to the environment. Organic farming is more labour intensive so you'll be supporting jobs and sometimes local businesses. And because it preserves biodiversity, ensuring greater food security, organic farming means you'll be getting a wider variety of fruit and vegetables.

An important aspect of overcoming menstrual health problems is to become an aware consumer. I have only given you a brief introduction. Because food is so central to your menstrual health, I encourage you to become more informed about the food you eat.

2. Food for Menstrual Health

The following dietary guidelines are ideal for continuing wellbeing for all women, but particularly for those who suffer from any menstrual problem including premenstrual syndrome (PMS), endometriosis and dysmenorrhoea, fibroids, cysts, PID and an irregular cycle. It's important to remember that each person's needs are unique. No one diet fits everyone, but there are some useful guidelines.

Many women ask me: "How long do I have to be on this diet?" This is like asking: "How long is a piece of string?" It's a difficult question for me to answer, partly because I would never recommend going back to a poor nutrient deficient diet. You may in the future be able to enjoy foods on the "to avoid" list, but they would be occasional rather than a regular feature of your diet. It also greatly depends on what your overall health is like. So how long you stay on the diet depends on each individual woman.

As a general guideline, you need to give yourself at least three months on your new diet to allow for any health changes. Give yourself longer, say five or six months, if you are a bit on again/off again with the diet.

No matter how small the changes you've made to your diet, you may have days when you can't do it. This is perfectly normal, so don't beat yourself up for eating inappropriate foods — enjoy eating them, and then continue again the next day with the healthier plan. Do it consciously, plan treats for yourself, rather than furtively react to that "damn diet". If life without chocolate, for instance, feels unbearable, treat yourself occasionally to a small amount of the best! Consider also buying organic chocolate with unrefined cane sugar — it's delicious. My only word of caution: try not to break the health rules in the few days before and during your period.

Foods that promote health

Whole foods and minimally processed foods. Examples of whole foods are brown rice rather than white rice, brown flour rather than white flour. Minimally processed foods include tofu and fermented foods such as miso and yoghurt.

Fresh food. I have a contract with myself not to eat food that's more than a day old. For example, I might make enough dinner so there's some left over for a lunch box the next day, but if I haven't eaten it by then I throw it away. It's important to avoid food that has gone mouldy, particularly if you have allergies. Remember to enjoy foods in season.

Organically and biodynamically produced food. Organically and biodynamically produced food is much tastier and contains more vitamins and minerals than conventionally produced food. Most importantly, it doesn't contain the pesticides, chemical fertilisers, growth hormones, antibiotics and vaccines that regular fruit, vegetables, meat, eggs and dairy products contain. Avoid genetically engineered food at all times. Buying certified organic food is one way to ensure you're not eating genetically engineered food.

The greatest possible variety. You're more likely to get the range of nutrients your body needs if you have a varied diet. You're also less likely to develop an allergy which can occur if you repeatedly eat the same foods.

Vegetables. Most vegies are rich in vitamins and minerals. Particularly good ones for women with menstrual problems are root vegies and the green leafy varieties. Make fresh vegetables the mainstay of your diet.

Whole grains and whole grain cereal. These include brown rice, corn, oats, rye, millet, buckwheat, quinoa, amaranth and wheat. Wheat can worsen bloating and gas, a sign that you could be allergic to it. In your quest for menstrual health, I would even go so far as to say that wheat be one of the foods you consider giving up first.

Legumes. These include lentils, kidney beans, azuki beans, chick peas, haricot beans, lima beans, black-eyed beans, black beans, split peas.

Seeds and nuts. Avoid peanuts and peanut butter, as well as pistachios, as they usually contain mould. Unlike meat and fish, beans, nuts and seeds are not complete proteins. However, by coupling them with a grain, you have a complete protein. You don't need to eat them in the same meal to get the benefit of the protein. It's important to store nuts, seeds, and their spreads, in the refrigerator to prevent them from becoming rancid. Eat nuts and seeds within a few weeks of purchase and only buy from shops where there's a high turnover of stock. Avoid stale nuts and seeds at all costs.

Fruits. Enjoy fruits that are seasonal. Fresh fruit is a good source of vitamins and fibre.

Oils. Use only cold-pressed, unrefined oils. Olive (virgin only) and sesame are the best for every day use. Avoid canola oil. Ideally buy oils in brown bottles, to minimise the deteriorating effects of light, and keep them in the refrigerator. Don't even think about buying the de-odourised, sanitised (hydrogenated) versions you find in supermarkets. Hydrogenation creates an immune damaging fat so these oils have no goodness left in them and may even be bad for you.

Essential fatty acids (EFAs). Essential for good health, EFAs are particularly important for women with menstrual problems. We need them for the formation of the "friendly" prostaglandins that help to ease cramping. Particularly rich sources of EFAs are flaxseed (linseed), evening primrose, raw goat's milk and the oil in fatty fish. Enjoy freshly ground linseed sprinkled on you food as an economical and easy way to get these nutrients.

Tofu. Made from soy beans, tofu is a good protein source. Soy beans are a source of plant oestrogens which may help relieve PMS symptoms by competing with your own level of oestrogen when it's too high. Tofu is not fermented, so if you have severe health problems or very poor digestion, avoid eating it.

Shoyu or tamari. These are fermented soya products made from water, salt and soya beans. Use as a salt substitute as it contains much less sodium.

Miso. A fermented soya bean paste, miso contains protein and helps fight fatigue. It's a great aid to digestion — as long as you don't boil the paste — and a good salt substitute.

Tempeh. An Indonesian food, tempeh is fermented soya beans (again!). It's very nutritious and an excellent protein product.

Although an acquired taste for some people it's worthwhile learning some tasty recipes.

Seaweeds. A powerhouse of minerals, vitamins and amino acids, seaweeds are an excellent source of iodine, calcium and iron in an easily assimilated form. Never mind diamonds being a girl's best friend, minerals are — seaweeds are a great way to ensure you get plenty of them! Seaweeds will help prevent damage to tissues from chemicals, heavy metals, and certain types of radioactivity; offset stress, boost stamina, and restore sexual interest (Weed,1989). Types of seaweed include nori, arame, kombu, wakame and Tasmanian float leaf. You can also buy kelp seaweed in tablet and powdered form, using the latter as a salt substitute if you wish.

Water. Essential for all chemical processes in your body, water also helps memory and flushes toxins from the body. I suspect that premenstrual headaches have a lot to do with dehydration. Start drinking more water from today, particularly in hot weather or if you exercise heavily. Because of the many chemicals used in our water supply, a water filter is essential. A reverse osmosis filter system is the best, but initially buy whatever you can afford. Or buy bottled water in clear plastic or glass bottles only.

The great soy debate

Although soy products, such as tofu and soy milk, are frequently touted as a great source of protein, and a panacea for the woes of menopause, some health practitioners believe soy products are too difficult to digest and should be avoided. Another complication is that soy beans were one of the first foods to be genetically engineered and for this reason alone I would encourage you to eat only organic or biodynamic soy.

The specific soy products I recommend are prepared using traditional methods such as soaking, long slow cooking and natural fermentation and are therefore OK. Other modern soy food, such as milk, cheese, and soy protein isolates used in some soy milks, protein supplements, baby formulas and many "instant" packaged foods, are prepared in high tech, high speed ways that denature the food. Research has found that these products are difficult to digest and can lead to deficiencies of zinc, calcium, B12, and vitamins A and D.

It's not necessary to eat soy products to have a healthy diet. If you don't like them don't force yourself. Listen to your body on this one!

3. The Menstrual Health Diet

The following table will help you work out specific ways to improve your diet. The foods listed in the "avoid or reduce" column are those foods that worsen menstrual health. Following the recommendations is particularly important if you experience menstrual symptoms; however, they are also useful for those women wishing to maintain wellbeing.

Avoid or reduce	Alternative
Dairy products: cow's milk and cheese, butter and butter spreads, yoghurt. (*Note:* women not experiencing menstrual difficulties can enjoy organic dairy products).	◆ Enjoy fermented organic and biodynamic products, such as yoghurt and cheese, that use unhomogenised milk.
Problem: ◆ Dairy products create a watery, bloated feeling or edema. This can worsen candida, and is implicated in a prolapsed uterus.	◆ Eat small amounts of goat's and sheep's milk products which are easier to digest than cow's. Unpasteurised goat's milk is also full of live enzymes, a nourishing food, that's more easily tolerated than other dairy products.
◆ Dairy products interfere with the absorption of magnesium, a mineral which is helpful for easing menstrual cramps, stabilising blood sugar levels and mood swings.	◆ Rice, almond or oat milk are good substitutes for cow's milk.
◆ They contribute to the production of series 2 prostaglandins (hormone like substances in the body) the "baddies" implicated in menstrual cramping. The "good" prostaglandins, series 1 and 3, which ease pain, are created by eating the healthy diet described here.	◆ Consider coming off dairy products altogether for at least three months, particularly if you have endometriosis. Later you may be able to enjoy them. ◆ Use seed and nut butter (e.g. tahini), and virgin olive oil instead of butter. Don't even consider margarine — throw out any tubs you have lurking in the fridge now.

Avoid or reduce

Yeasted breads and bakery products: commercial cakes, biscuits and pastries.

Problem:

◆ Yeast contributes to candida

◆ White flour acidifies the body and in turn leaches it of minerals

◆ Often made using hydrogenated oils.

Alternative

◆ Eat organic sourdough wholewheat bread. Some sourdoughs may contain a little yeast, so read the label carefully.

◆ Even better try a wheat-free sourdough bread or rice cakes.

◆ Minimise your consumption of breads, pasta and cakes altogether, and replace with small amounts of whole grains such as rice or millet.

◆ If life without cakes and cookies feels too miserable, try your health food store for the occasional sweet treat — naturally sweetened, and using cold pressed oils or butter. Although butter is on the "to avoid" list because it's too rich for your liver, it's much safer than the trans-fat/hydrogenated oils and is therefore preferable. Consider making your own sweet treats from one of the many excellent whole food cookery books on the market.

Avoid or reduce

Meat: beef, organ meats such as liver and kidneys, pork, lamb, chicken and meat products, such as sausages or hot dogs, and all deli meats which may contain nitrate preservatives.

Problem:

◆ Opinions vary on meat. Some health experts say all meat is bad, while others say we do need a little.

◆ Meat is difficult to digest and may lead to worsened pain and PMS.

◆ Non-organically produced meat is full of toxins from antibiotics, vaccines, hormones and pesticides.

◆ The chemicals in our environment get transported in the food chain through animal fats.

◆ Too much meat increases the body's demand for minerals.

Alternative

◆ I suggest eating meat no more than three times a week. Giving it up altogether even for a short time may be necessary for some of you, particularly if you have endometriosis and general cramping.

◆ Always eat lots of vegetables and fruit if you eat meat.

◆ At the very least don't eat animal fat.

◆ Best of all, only eat organically produced meat, minimising the fat.

◆ Eat instead deep ocean fish and occasional organic free range chicken. Don't even look at battery chicken except to take a stance for stopping the inhumane treatment of these birds.

◆ It's essential to only eat organ meats that are organically produced.

◆ Only ever eat organic free range eggs.

◆ Chicken soup made from the bones is also very nourishing.

◆ Don't forget the great vegetable sources of protein mentioned.

Avoid or reduce

Caffeinated drinks (coffee, tea and cola drinks) decaffeinated coffee

Problem:

◆ Caffeine depletes the body of B vitamins.

◆ It contributes to anxiety and irritability and worsens mood swings.

◆ Decaffeinated coffee contains solvents and even if it's water processed there are other inflammatory alkaloids.

◆ Caffeine may have an adverse effect on your fertility.

Alternative

◆ Unroasted or roasted dandelion root coffee is good for the liver and digestion.

◆ Grain-based beverages, such as Caro or Echo are safe substitutes for coffee.

◆ Ginger tea is excellent for fatigue. Bancha tea with a drop of shoyu and some grated ginger is also a great pick-me-up.

◆ Try also the wide variety of herbal teas. The mineral rich nettle tea is good for the kidneys and adrenals (the glands that sit on top of your kidneys and form part of your endocrine system) — a true friend to women!

Avoid or reduce

Alcohol

Problem:

◆ Alcohol depletes the body of minerals and B vitamins.

◆ It's toxic to the liver.

◆ It makes candida worse.

Alternative

◆ Drink no more than two glasses of wine, diluted with mineral water, a week.

◆ Fresh vegetable or fruit juice. Go very easy on fruit juice as it has a high sugar content — dilute it with purified water or mineral water.

◆ Consider giving up alcohol altogether and develop the water drinking habit.

Avoid or reduce

Refined sugar (sucrose), cane sugar, molasses, artificial sweeteners, soft drinks

Problem

◆ Sucrose and artificial sweeteners, such as aspartamine, nutrasweet and saccharin, are "empty" foods — they have no nutrient value and so are potentially bad for you. Sugar enters the blood stream too quickly, upsetting your blood sugar levels, stressing your adrenals. In the long run refined sugar makes you more fatigued and depletes you of minerals and B complex vitamins. It also contributes to premenstrual crankiness and fatigue. As your overall diet improves you may find your sugar cravings decrease.

◆ Soft drinks are full of either refined sugar or artificial sweeteners and are to be avoided all costs. Far from quenching your thirst they will dehydrate your body.

◆ The more sugar you eat, the more you will crave it.

Alternative

◆ Use rice or barley malt and sugar free jams.

◆ Use stevia, a very sweet herb, in place of sugar.

◆ Pear or apple juice concentrate, and dried fruits such as dates, are good baking sweeteners as the natural sugar enters the blood stream more slowly and therefore is much gentler on the body.

◆ Complex carbohydrates such as brown rice, wholemeal bread and oats can reduce your sugar craving. Try also baked pumpkin and sweet potato.

◆ Honey and maple syrup as a very occasional treat are OK if you're desperate!

Avoid or reduce	Alternative
Chocolate *Problem:* ◆ Chocolate contains refined sugar, which contributes to mood swings and breast tenderness. It also contains caffeine. ◆ Because it contains magnesium (good for cramping and mood swings) and the mood enhancer amino acid phenylalanine, you can understand why you might have such an intense craving just before bleeding. Alas, the other ingredients preclude it as a helpful food source!	◆ Unsweetened carob is a member of the legume family and high in calcium. You can buy carob in chunk form as a substitute for a chocolate bar or as a powder to use in baking and drinks. Beware — some brands of carob "chocolate" contain sugar. Avoid these! Read the labels carefully — there are some tasty brands that don't contain sugar. ◆ Although organic choc is still chocolate, it has a lot more going for it than the regular stuff. And it's expensive which may act as a tiny brake on overindulgence! The odd mouthful in those chocolate crises may do a lot for your psyche without too much upset to your body.

Avoid or reduce

Free-flowing salt and high sodium foods (bouillon, commercial salad dressings and tomato sauces, salty snack foods)

Problem

◆ These foods worsen bloating and fluid retention.

◆ Regular free flowing salt bought in supermarkets contains additives — so avoid it!

◆ The added sugar, hydrogenated oils, preservatives and food colouring in commercial sauces, dressings and snack foods are just further flak for your body to deal with.

Alternative

◆ You may need a little salt — I recommend mineral rich coarse sea salt from your health food shop. It looks grey and lumpy, and will definitely not flow through your salt shaker!

◆ Try seasoning your foods with herbs, a little shoyu or miso.

◆ You can buy good quality tomato sauce, mayonnaise and dressings, without additives, at health food shops — always check labels carefully.

Making Life Easier

* Think about adding new foods to your diet before removing the less supportive ones.

* If you eat a lot of the foods on the "avoid" list, **don't** come off them suddenly.

* Change one thing at a time. Start with what's easiest for you e.g. drinking more water.

* Relax and enjoy what you eat while being honest with yourself and tuning into your body's specific needs. If you run on a diet of coffee and sugar, both addictive substances, it will take you a little time to identify your body's genuine needs from an addictive craving.

* Be especially careful about sticking to the healthy diet in the second half of your menstrual cycle, particularly the week before you bleed and during bleeding.

* Make sure you have plenty of nutritious but tasty snacks available at all times to stop the "munchies" from forcing you down to the corner shop.

* Don't shop when you're hungry.

* Get a good wholefood, sugar free, recipe book and/or go to some health oriented cookery lessons. Any new diet can be time consuming, and some of the ingredients of the one I have recommended take time to prepare — beans and grains will not be hurried!

★ Chew your food really well. The first stage of digestion, in particular with carbohydrates, begins in the mouth. The action of chewing also helps to stimulate hydrochloric acid in the stomach which is essential for protein digestion.

★ Eat when you're feeling calm. If you're upset, wait until your feelings have settled.

★ Although some oil in the diet is necessary, avoid fried and oily foods, particularly around menstruation.

★ Avoid extremely hot or extremely cold food as it may cause indigestion.

★ At menstruation, eat lightly and prepare easily digestable foods such as soups. For example, one pot "soupy" dishes with some grain, vegies and some beans or a little fish simmered together for a while with the addition of some herbs or a little fresh ginger is perfect.

★ Eat defrosted food that you've prepared yourself, rather than packaged pre-prepared food. This is infinitely preferable to finding yourself starving and rushing out for pizza because there's nothing easy on hand to prepare.

★ Avoid aluminium and copper cookware — use only glass or stainless steel.

★ Minimise use of canned food.

★ Always read labels assiduously — you need to become your own watch dog. Avoid all foods containing synthetic colouring and additives.

To eat raw food or not?

Traditional Chinese Medicine does **not** recommend eating raw food the week before and during your menstruation. It takes more energy to digest and is cooling on the body. Of course, eating foods that cool the body are, for instance, important during the hot days of summer. However, generally when we menstruate, and particularly if we have problems, eating more "warming", easily digestible foods is, overall, very nourishing and supportive for the body.

In the Western naturopathic traditions, raw food is seen as A Good Thing. I come from a macrobiotic (Asian) approach to food, where everything is cooked. Today I'm drawn to the Western naturopathic model — I eat at least 75 per cent of my diet as raw and feel fantastic. Cooking destroys enzymes which are essential for health. While our bodies produce their own enzymes, this is not enough if you prefer cooked food. Listen to your own instincts on what feels right to you. If your digestion is very vulnerable it might be good to go easy on raw food initially. Lightly cooking the food does not destroy all its nutrients and sometimes makes them more available to the body.

Menstruation, the World and You

"TO WOMAN THE CREATOR HAS GIVEN THE SACRED
CHARGE TO PURIFY AND REDREAM THE WORLD DURING
HER MOONTIME"

Mooncircle teachings

1.   *Acting for the World*

The world moves us and we move the world. We are not isolated self contained units. We are connected in countless ways to the world. Our wellbeing is the world's wellbeing and vice versa. Think of you and the world as one.

Menstrual disturbance, as with any symptom or illness, has its locus in a particular body but speaks for the time and place in which that body is situated. As you approach your body in the manner I'm suggesting you'll be responding to the promptings of the world. It's an inescapable fact that you'll be working for the world in some way.

Menstruation is a window of opportunity, a gap through which you get to peek into the inner workings and state of your body and soul. This window of opportunity is also an opening to the dreams of the world. Your symptoms are a call from the world to do things differently and to make it a better place. To treat illness as though it were an isolated phenomenon, unconnected both to your personal future and to the condition of the world, is short sighted.

The trouble for many of us at menstruation is that "the world" often feels all too demanding. We'd be happiest if we could stop it for a while, step off and find ourselves a snug cocoon where all faxes, phones, mobiles, modems or otherwise were banned. This cocoon wouldn't exist on a map — we could find it only because of our brilliant homing device at menstruation for solitude and peace!

At menstruation it's as though the world is using the opportunity of our vulnerability to speak to us of its own condition and needs. If you approach your symptoms by trying to get yourself back to "normal" and restoring the status quo you are betraying the world, not just yourself. This betrayal will consistently sabotage your attempts at finding lasting relief.

How do we manage then when those around us are not eager for us to drop our usual ebullient, productive, and glamorous selves regardless of our vitally important inner impulses to be difficult, daggy and slothful? How do we manage when we no longer fit in **nicely**?

To do this you may initially need to draw on your amazing talent for multi tasking: resting while still having to go to work or look after children; switching off from the world while still being plugged in to the task at hand. Most of us don't have the luxury of not having to earn a living, and our children's needs don't suddenly disappear when we bleed. Yet there are ways to accommodate and work around this conundrum. The first step is to feel OK about following your changing rhythm and to visualise what you would like for yourself. Always remember that menstruation becomes the opportunity for examining and reordering the life that is yours.

The Truth Speaker

How many times have you been told your passionate feelings about something are not rational, and therefore not relevant? You're told that because you're full of feeling you're no longer capable of making "intelligent" responses. This is the dominant approach in many cultures — one that is focused on the "rational", on abstract reasoning. It's a tyranny that has been imposed on us as individuals and the world as a whole. It's a one sided and reductionist approach — confining us within a limited world view. It's an approach that turns us against the world. It makes us try to fit into what's already known — and stops us from allowing the unknown to teach and guide us.

The way into the unknown is through the rich play of our sensory experience. We need to learn how to trust our feelings and senses as signs of things not yet known to the rational mind. We're being extended beyond the known, and asked to be with, to act in the name of something beyond ourselves, but which we must still think of as somehow us. It involves allowing ourselves to experience fully and with awareness the feelings that come to us. It's this act of feeling that will inform us. To leap to "rational" interpretation and explanation without engaging with the intelligence of the experience itself deadens vitality — our own and the world's. It leads to a dead end.

Sometimes it reminds me of a dog tracking a scent. The dog is always totally involved and through that activity is led somewhere. Our feelings and sense of things are like the picking up of scents laid down by the earth to lead us on and open us to knowledge and wisdom. Our feelings and intuitions are immediate, bypassing preconceptions to grasp the whole.

At menstruation right brain talents are in the ascendancy — that's when we most diverge from the dominant cultural ethos of "cool and detached is best". Regard menstruation as a liberation, a chance to know the world more easily and directly. Go slowly with it — this way of accessing knowledge won't be rushed. It requires all those dreamy, fluid imaginings that you so specialise in when you bleed.

In some cultures, women would stop all their regular activities and retreat from the community at menstruation. As Lara Owen points out, in societies comfortable with women's power this retreat was seen as a positive and sacred process. In cultures where the opposite was true she was made to retreat because she was considered a danger to the community (Owen, 1993). Her presence could spoil the crops, spoil a man's chances of succeeding in the hunt, and make him impotent to boot. She was also generally considered bad news for any cooking or brewing.

Menstrual practices were originally put in place by women — while they may have later been interpreted in a negative light, women were still the authors of the process. But whether configured positively or negatively the stories are still referring to a great power.

How can these stories be useful to us today particularly when it's impossible for us to retreat in such a manner except in rare circumstances? Does that mean that we're doing ourselves and the world an enormous disservice? Maybe we are dangerous to the community, maybe we do spoil the cooking. Before you knock me on the head for apparently having just set women's position back a few hundred years, I'm not suggesting we are capable of jinxing others. We are capable of exerting greater power at this time to influence the world.

I believe it is dangerous to ignore our needs and feelings. Menstruation's talents don't want to be wasted on everyday stuff, and cooking and tending to others is everyday stuff. I know several women who don't cook well during the menstrual upheaval. How many of you have silly accidents and feel you jar with everything around you?

Too right you disturb — there's a part of you mightily pissed off about wasting your visionary and regenerative skills by continuing on the same as before! Trying not to cause disturbance is like trying to stop the force of change. It's wasting something valuable in yourself.

I have often reflected on those people who choose to retreat from the world as a way of life, usually as part of their spiritual work. I now recognise that this work is vital to the stability of the world. There is some knowledge you can only access by being in that kind of space. The world would be an even madder place than it already is if it were not for these people's capacity to hold the place of solitude and silence. If you're feeling irresponsible for wanting to drop out for a while, remember Heraclitus who said "Even sleepers are workers and collaborators in what goes on in the universe" (Hall, 1980, p.xiii)!

A menstruating woman's retreat was regarded as healing for the whole community. Owen tells us that the Cherokee recognise menstruating women as "performing a function of cleansing and centering not only for herself but also for her family, and therefore the whole tribe." (Owen, 1998, p.167). She visions for the community. She is Truth Speaker, doing the work of priestess and speaker of oracles. Here is our work for the world — I believe the real danger lies in avoiding that work. Avoidance will only contribute to our menstrual difficulties.

There are a number of things you can do. One is to stand up for Menstrual Retreat or at the very least a Menstrual Slowdown. You can also learn to wield your menstrual power in your particular environment. For example, instead of riding over your feelings and need for slowness, put those qualities to good use. If you find yourself crying, see this as a way of softening the unfeelingness that exists in the world. Notice yourself soften and sense what has opened to you through the crying.

Use your sensitivity to read beyond the obvious and see into the depths of issues. Influence others with the wisdom of your slowness. Listen to yourself. If you're crabby in the premenstruum, don't apologise — bring it out! Be critical and stand up for yourself. I remember one women who capitalised on her premenstrual aggro by sorting out difficult issues in the workplace — particularly when she had to deal with men who had more authority than she had. She wasn't fazed in the premenstruum!

Find ways to have more solitude even if you're at work —

you'll be achieving things in a different way and will allow creative ideas to flood in. There'll come a time when women's visionary skill at menstruation and after menopause will be used in research and development projects! So cruise with those dreamy, intuitive states and notice what serendipitous things occur when you're not always pushing yourself, not always "on the ball". Capitalise on that cleaning and sorting bug that seems to hit many of us premenstrually...all those long standing petty little tasks suddenly get done.

Sometimes a menstruating woman acts like a lightening conductor, picking up the unexpressed charge in the atmosphere around her because of her enhanced permeability. This means you may be feeling things that are not entirely personal to you. You may be the oracle for the unspoken and unattended issues in your workplace or wider environment. These are everyone's concerns and not just yours. But you may be feeling them for others, particularly if those people are not in touch with their feeling sides.

Feeling for the world

Virginia experiences an overwhelming sense of responsibility to act for the world. What she feels most passionate about is the environment " ... what we're doing to it ... injustice, prejudice, the dumbing down of society. I care too much!" She feels angry at what's going on and angry with herself for not doing enough. On around day 21 of her 28 day cycle, it comes crashing in on her with even greater intensity. The rage, mostly self directed, startles her with its force.

Although premenstrual disturbance has been Virginia's companion for a number of years, it's getting worse — she feels it's beating her. As a freelance writer her life has its fair share of stresses. Sometimes it's worry over meeting deadlines from too much work. At other times work is lean and she worries about paying her bills. Despite the roller coaster ride, she feels she's on the road she wants to be on — it's just not happening fast enough. Her inner critic is exacting and, in that premenstrual phase, unrelenting in its demands on her.

Coupled with her fiercely driven energy to make a difference in the world is an incredible sensitivity. A capacity to enter altered states and feel the presence of spirits. After she has begun to bleed she can also feel herself detaching and going off in her internal space. It's like "being let off the leash to wander in the cosmos. I'm happy to let go and want to see what's sent back." It's an incredibly creative space.

Even at her best times Virginia wrestles with big forces in her — in the limenal space of the premenstruum it simply becomes too much. Like many of us, she needs to be a little kinder with herself, to validate what she has done, rather than focusing solely on her failings. It's vitally important for women like Virginia, who feel a deep calling to serve the world, to take great care of their menstrual sensitivity. Awareness of the cycle is critical so they are prepared for that extra vulnerability and can do what they need to do to minimise distress.

Like many of the women in this book, Virginia is rocked by the "old knowing" which she must grow into. As she learns better self care, she'll learn to channel that force. She will realise her dream to become an activist and ally for the world, without suffering too much stress.

Sometimes disturbance, such as rage, is fuelled by social injustice. Your rage may come from your capacity to "see" the injustice and you are called upon to be the Truth Speaker. I also believe there is an archetypal rage at work in women. A rage that resides in the very core of our beings handed on from generation to generation, a rage at the injustices that have been meted out to women through the centuries. I only have to think of the Burning Times in the Middle Ages when it is estimated many thousands, maybe millions, of women were burnt ostensibly for being witches, to feel anger stir in me. Witches could be any independent, free thinking women who were also sometimes healers, midwives or heretics. They were persecuted and burned by the Christian Church who believed only men should have those powers and abilities.

And injustices continue to be perpetrated against women — domestic violence, inequity in the workplace, genital mutilation and sexual exploitation, to name a few. These global concerns can fuel our personal upset. Recognising this may help you understand and handle your personal upheavals. Even better, you can use this rage as a force for changing the world, the way Janice does (see her story in Restoring Imagination).

Restoring rhythm

Our modern lifestyle coerces us into overriding natural rhythms. We have the option to stay switched on 24 hours a day, 365 days a year. Working around the clock, playing around the clock. Our needs instantly gratified. It's enormously intoxicating. Nothing can stop us it seems. Buzzy and great though it may feel, it's unsustainable. It's rhythmless. And loss of rhythm is death. The rhythm of nature — the seasons, the days, our bodies — are the basis for life. It's the movement between different states that keeps us alive, vital and resilient.

The changing seasons of the womb are what help to keep it healthy. To try to cauterise, or override, one part of our cycle is to damage a natural system of generation and regeneration. This is true for all rhythms. To take a stand for rhythm is to take a stand for the very basis of our existence.

The destruction to the environment wrought by our high speed living which seeks always to find ways to dominate nature rather than work with it, concerns me. I like to imagine that in our slowing down at menstruation, nature too might rest. In understanding our own need for rhythm we are respecting nature's rhythm.

We could recognise, for example, that ancient practice of letting soil rest. Crops were rotated and fields in turn allowed to lie fallow for one season. This was not seen as a waste of land but good husbandry, a necessity to restore the vitality of the soil. Instead we now flog the soil to death with more and more fertilisers and pesticides in the same way we flog our bodies with coffee, sugar and drugs to keep hyped and on the move. Like the soil that eventually becomes so denuded nothing more will grow in it, we too will wear down our own physical and creative vitality.

The world needs more from us than just rest. It needs a restoring of the sacred and of the power of women. Remember, the bleeding is our Sabbath. At the Sabbath, or holy days, we go to the sacred places to pray and make offerings to the Divine and give thanks to the world. Yet, we have largely placed all our religious practice in the hands and buildings of the established religions. We have forgotten that our own bodies are entry points through which we can walk to touch the numinous. If women collectively used menstruation as sacred time we would unleash enormous psychic forces.

Some societies, particularly Australian Aborigines, believed that if women were allowed to menstruate together the world would be overwhelmed by floods and fires and would come to an end (Shuttle and Redgrove, 1995). That's some power! No wonder some men get edgy around menstruation and no wonder we have to be distracted from it! Rejection of our menstrual cycle, and menstruation itself, means we're at war with our bodies, and therefore ourselves. So much energy tied up. Understanding and acceptance of the power of the cycle, liberates that energy, opening us to power and to the world.

Collective menstrual power, I suspect, would rebel against that all consuming economic rationalist monster reducing life to a balance sheet, and human beings to nothing more than robotic creatures streamlined to maximise efficiency. Try as we do to control, soul life will always out. The sacred will reply, the earth rebel. The more "efficiency" we try to impose on the world at the expense of human qualities and natural systems, the more distress, chaos and environmental degradation occurs. Our so called efficiency ends up looking more like endless damage control from the fallout of soulless planning.

Knowledge of the deep transformative powers of the feminine make it impossible to tolerate the nightmare that is daily unfolding on our planet. This knowledge humbles the ego which, in its determination to only serve itself, ironically can only end in self destruction.

2. Acting for the Environment

We are in dire straits. In our industrialised high-tech-throw-away-life we refuse to recognise that we are part of nature. It's imperative that we listen to the world's aches and pains. Full scale emergencies already exist including water shortages that hamper developing countries, land degradation that reduce soil fertility and agricultural potential, and irreversible destruction of the tropical rainforest. Launching the *Global Environment Outlook 2000* report Klaus Topfer, the executive director of the UN environment program, said that to reverse environmental degradation, the conspicuous overconsumption by the world's rich countries must be cut by 90%.

We are now paying the price, including damage to our health, for disrupting natural systems. Your endometriosis, fibroid, excessive blood, pain, premenstrual anguish, polycystic ovaries are all directly linked to increasing environmental pollution.

Research from Germany found that women with endometriosis had high levels of PCBs (polychlorinated biphenyls) and dioxins in their bodies. Chemicals such as pesticides, plastics and heavy metals act as "oestrogen mimickers". They are able to attach themselves to oestrogen receptor sites in the body thereby upsetting the oestrogen/progesterone balance and consequently the natural synergy of a woman's body. We are literally swimming in a sea of synthetic oestrogens which are damaging not only to human bodies but to nature as well. This phenomenon is known as the feminisation of nature. Ironic if you think about it — the feminine has snuck in the back door as a major disruptor! If the effects were not so catastrophic it would be funny.

Through every day exposure to toxic chemicals and electromagnetic radiation, our body's ability to repair itself is being seriously zapped. There are chemicals in the water that comes out of our taps and in the food we buy — meat laced with carcinogenic and oestrogenic substances, vegetables and fruit sprayed with toxic pesticide. They are in the everyday technology we use including microwave ovens, televisions, electric blankets, electric clocks, computers, mobile phones, fax machines. There are chemicals in household cleaners, pest sprays, garden fertilisers, clothes, furnishings, skin and hair products, makeup, perfumes, washing powders, paints, plastics, newspapers, magazines and books. Outside the home we have pollution from cars and trucks, aeroplanes, polluting industries and chemicalised agribusiness. The accumulative drip drip drip of all these stressors plays havoc with human physiology, with effects that include cancer, infertility, immune suppression, birth defects, and still births.

To heal and maintain wellbeing it's **absolutely essential** to minimise pollutants in our personal life and attend to the environment as a whole. Remember, if the planet goes under, we all go with it. The political will to make change at present is almost nonexistent. We cannot afford to wait for governments to act but instead we need to take action ourselves through the everyday decisions we make. Don't underestimate the power of your individual acts to make a difference. Although you may only be focusing on your own immediate environment, you'll be helping your family, friends and co-workers. And the slow drip drip drip of your collective refusal to support polluting products and practices will add up to a big "yes" for the environment. Consumer power is enormous.

With time, as you clean up your environment along with doing all the other health practices I recommend, you'll find yourself carried along by a strong wave of well being. This might inspire you to take bigger steps that involve support for environmental organisations, social action, or a reorganisation of your whole life to one based on restorative principles. Regardless of whether you suffer health problems, I urge you to read further on environmental issues. The following points are a starting place to make changes in your personal environment.

Food — the danger	*What you can do*
Food can be spoiled by thoughtless packaging, or cooking it in aluminium or enamel cookware. Food that has been cooked or defrosted in a microwave can cause changes in the blood. This process is indicative of similar processes found in cancer (Best, 2000).	◆ Avoid canned food and plastic packaging. At the very least remove food from the packaging as soon as possible. ◆ Store food in glass containers. ◆ Use cloth and paper bags for storing vegetables. ◆ Try cellophane bags for storing or short term freezing only. ◆ Avoid aluminium and copper cookware, and avoid cooking or storing food in aluminium foil. ◆ Ideally use glass cookware. ◆ Avoid tetra packs which are lined with aluminium. ◆ Don't microwave your food. It's especially critical that you don't microwave children's food. ◆ Only drink or cook with filtered water, ideally filtered using the reverse osmosis system. ◆ Never eat processed breakfast cereals (they contain solvent remnants) and avoid processed foods wherever possible.

Food — the danger	*What you can do (cont)*
	◆ Eat organic and biodynamic foods, and avoid genetically modified and irradiated food.

Your body — the danger

Skin and hair products are a minefield of synthetic chemicals. Most of the chemicals that go into our toiletries are also the harsh toxic chemicals used in industry. For example, popylene glycol found in makeup, hair care products, deodorants and aftershave, is also the main ingredient in anti freeze and brake fluid. Polyethylene glycol found in most skin cleansers, is a caustic used to dissolve grease (Thomas, 1999). Because the skin absorbs everything it's as good as eating it — and of course in the case of lipstick you literally are! So stop and think before you pile it on.

The good news is, the healthier you become the less you will need to lather your body with potions. Beauty is an inside job. Environmental pollution is what's aging us the most. Clean up your lifestyle, your personal environment as much as you can, and your diet, and you'll start looking utterly gorgeous. Always remember that manufacturing of makeup is still an imperfect process, so avoid using it as much as possible.

What you can do

◆ Use plant based beauty products, including perfumes, rather than petrochemically based ones. Listing some natural ingredients doesn't mean the product is all natural — so beware.

◆ Read labels carefully. Avoid ingredients such as sodium lauryl/laureth sulfate, talc, mineral oil, aluminium, glycol, and ones containing the letters "prop" e.g. propyl, propamine, isopropyl, propanol and propylene.

◆ Telephone the manufacturer and ask them to explain the ingredients and where they come from.

◆ Avoid using foundation as it prevents your skin breathing.

◆ Use toothpaste that is free of fluoride, sugar and sodium lauryl sulphate.

◆ Avoid hair dyes, especially dark colours.

◆ Use only biodegradable low allergenic formula washing powders and washing up liquids free of unnecessary colourings and fragrances.

194 The Wild Genie

Your body — the danger	*What you can do (cont)*
	◆ Avoid having your clothes dry cleaned. If you must have this done, air the item of clothing outside for three days afterwards before wearing it. ◆ Avoid antiperspirants and deodorants, especially those containing aluminium. If you wear natural fibres you'll sweat less. Body odour will also decrease as you clean up your diet and lifestyle. The best underarm deodoriser is a dusting of plain old bicarbonate of soda. If the powder stings or burns, it means it has been contaminated during manufacture and should be thrown out and replaced with a different brand. ◆ Stop smoking and avoid passive smoking. ◆ Avoid mercury fillings. You could consider having existing mercury fillings removed — make sure this is done by a dentist fully versed in the protocol and who has a completely mercury free practice. Having your amalgam fillings removed is not a procedure to enter into lightly although it may be necessary if your health is very poor. Read widely and ask questions before you make a decision. ◆ Avoid x-rays. ◆ Avoid oral contraceptives and wearing IUDs. ◆ Minimise or avoid using tampons especially if you suffer period pain.

Your home — the danger

You might be thinking, or hoping, that your home is a haven from the pollutants of the world. Alas! The modern home is an unhealthy place which can be polluted from cleaning agents and polishes, pesticides, lead based paints, synthetic carpets and chemical treatments in furniture. The good news is you can turn it into a safer haven.

What you can do

◆ Use only "green" cleaning products. Check logos to ensure they have been tested and validated by the appropriate government agency.

◆ For all general cleaning and laundry, try old fashioned products such as bicarbonate of soda for sinks, refrigerators, baths and toilets. White vinegar can be used as a disinfectant.

◆ Avoid all pesticides but if you do need a thorough pest proofing of your home, use only pyrethrum type compounds.

◆ Practice co-existence with insect life where possible. Put all food away and keep surfaces clean. To get rid of cockroaches try leaving out a bowl of beer — they'll at least die happy!

◆ You can buy non toxic pest control products, including treatment for animal fleas. If you have a flea infestation, vacuum thoroughly for ten consecutive days, replace the vacumm bag each time, throwing out the used one right away.

◆ If you need a pest exterminator, contract an ecologically sound one. They will often be able to give you advice about safely minimising pests in your home.

◆ Keep soft plastic out of your life as much as possible e.g. plastic bags of any kind, cling film, bubble wrap. Check every cupboard, it's surprising how much can be lurking. Also check the boot and inside of your car.

Your home — the danger	*What you can do (cont)*
	◆ Avoid aerosols and propellent sprays of any kind.
	◆ Avoid cooking on gas, or using gas heaters, and consider changing to electric.
	◆ Keep your home well aired at all times, especially the bathroom, to prevent build up of mould.
	◆ Have live plants throughout the house to absorb pollution.
	◆ Use a chlorine filter on the bath and shower heads, particularly the latter. You can absorb much more chlorine through breathing in the steam than through drinking.
	◆ Use ionisers, especially at night when sleeping. Place the ioniser close to an open window to blow the negative ions through the room. Or buy two and place on either side of the bed. For maximum effect have several ionisers in the one room.
	◆ When doing any renovations only use ecologically sound products (paint, stripper, varnishes) and beware of breathing in dust from the renovations.
	◆ If you have a choice avoid carpets, enjoy (naturally!) polished wooden floors with rugs made from natural fibres.
	◆ If you're a keen gardener, learn about organic and permaculture techniques to avoid use of pesticides, herbicides. Your garden will be healthier and happier as well!

Your workplace — the danger

If you work in an office you're likely to experience the same hazards as in the home — toxic cleaning agents, synthetic carpeting, and outgasing from furniture and technical equipment. Most offices are also sealed environments devoid of fresh air. And if you work in the city, the fresh air you get at lunch time is also polluted. Arrgghhh!! You may also work in industries where there is a high use of chemicals, for example if you're a hairdresser, photographer, beautician, agricultural worker, chemical worker, textile and leather worker or if you work in the car manufacturing and repair industry. Those working with electronics and semi conductors, food workers, workers in manufacturing and printing, glass and pottery, and hospital and health care staff are all at risk. The products used in these fields may affect your immune system and therefore overall health, including menstrual and reproductive health (Naish and Roberts, 1996)

What you can do

◆ Learn basic information about workplace chemicals and their toxic effects.

◆ Meticulously follow all safety precautions.

◆ Keep workspaces as well ventilated as possible.

◆ Consider changing your job.

◆ Use ionisers and live plants — the peace lily and spider plant absorb air pollution well, particularly around computers.

◆ Don't stand over photocopiers when they're in use.

City living — the danger

Living in cities can be a health hazard — it's almost impossible to avoid breathing in large quantities of polluting chemicals. So it's all the more important that you maintain lots of healthy practices such as exercise and a good diet.

Sadly, living in the country may not always be the paradise we imagine because of the pervasive use of agribusiness chemicals such as pesticides, fertilisers and fungicides.

What you can do

◆ Focus on controlling the things you can control.

◆ If you own a car, use it less often to minimise your contribution to air pollution.

◆ If you drive, avoid heavy traffic, tunnels and using underground or enclosed parking.

◆ Keep windows closed in heavy traffic and enclosed areas.

◆ Consider using an ioniser in the car.

◆ Minimise how frequently you fill your car with petrol and try to avoid breathing in the fumes as much as possible.

◆ Avoid exercising in heavy traffic areas.

◆ Avoid other people's cigarette smoke and perfumes.

Electro Magnetic Radiation (EMR) — the danger

Radiation comes from x-rays, microwaves, high voltage power lines, televisions, VDUs, mobile phones and all electrical devices. Although it's difficult to avoid, particularly in some workplaces, you can minimise electrical activity in your home. For example, you might think electric clocks and hair dryers are fairly benign but their EMR effect is very strong.

What you can do

◆ Don't keep an electric clock by your bed.

◆ Avoid electric blankets, or if you must have one, switch it off before going to sleep.

◆ Avoid hair dryers.

◆ Unplug all appliances that are not in use.

◆ Avoid locating beds and chairs close to domestic sources of EMR such as electricity meters and televisions.

◆ Use an ioniser especially when working at a computer. Either place the ioniser at eye level on top of the computer or buy two and put them on either side of you for a stereophonic effect. Never use just one ioniser on one side of you, as it will unbalance the body.

◆ Place plants around your computer, especially the spider plant and peace lily.

◆ Have regular epsom salt baths to help "cleanse" yourself of the effects of EMRs. Have plenty of contact with nature and the earth, even touching the plants in your office.

◆ Move away from your computer screen when involved in other activities.

◆ Turn off your computer when not in use.

◆ Try sipping water throughout the day, especially if you work at a computer or other electronic equipment.

The voice of Aphrodite

Dressed to kill and exquisitely made up, Monica sailed into one of my workshops. She looked beautiful. She also had health problems. Suffering from endometriosis, she also had interstitial cystitis, bowel problems and would faint at her period. Now, 34 years old, and very reliant on painkillers, she has been in out of hospital for the past sixteen years.

I could see that the kind of care Monica lavished on her body was going to have to change. Presenting the information about environmental influences on health, in particular beauty products, made me nervous. "But I'm an artist. This is one way I express my art!" protested Monica. I was on her side. But for her to maintain this form of her art she needed to find products that would not harm her body. While she always insists on products that have not been tested on animals, there is currently very little makeup on the market that is not harmful.

Although these things themselves don't directly cause endometriosis or other conditions, they do contribute to toxicity in the body which in turn leads to a wearing away of the body's resilience and ultimately to illness. Toxic toiletries are a particular problem for women like Monica, whose immune systems are already weak. Perhaps those of you who want to wear makeup will be the activists demanding beauty without toxicity.

Apart from makeup being a form of expression for her, it's also a protective mask. Her brave face. Nights of insomnia and days of pain take their toll. "They can't tell at work if I'm suffering when I wear the makeup. I can face the world a little better with it." Her long term poor health has taken on a kind of normality. A number of personal tragedies have also drained her emotionally, stretching her inner resources even further. Although she is aware of the need to do some inner work to learn to love her body/self more, she doesn't yet feel up to this task. The makeup provides a temporary place of refuge.

Because she cares about beauty, perhaps her Work in the world can be about taking a stand for Beauty.

3. *Managing Work*

To take care of our physical and inner needs without jeopardising our work is quite a challenge. If you're strong and healthy you might be able to ride over your inner needs. Not so if you're physically vulnerable. But why would you want to ignore your inner imperatives, even if you're healthy? If we work seven days a week, with no day off; if we don't allow some shift in the rhythm of our work to attend to our internal needs, we are likely to end up feeling cheated and exhausted.

Our uteruses have often been seen as a liability in the workplace. It looks like menstruation is indeed something we could well do without if we want to hold our ground with men and get ahead in the world. It's depressing to recognise that all the qualities that humanise, build intimacy and nourish the sacred are the ones that are less valued in the workplace. In many workplaces, if we reveal these aspects of ourselves we risk being ridiculed or not taken seriously.

It's untenable for me to suppress these qualities. And I can see it's untenable in all my psychotherapy clients, women and men alike, many of whom hold down (a telling phrase!) highly professional jobs. I think it's untenable for all of us — whether we'll admit to it or not. It's a shallow victory if to get ahead at work we must cauterise our soul life. We need an evolution in the world of work that builds social capital along with bank accounts. And where making money is a wholly owned subsidiary of making soul!

In some countries, such as Japan, women are entitled to take a day off for menstruation. Rarely in Japan is this taken up. Women's position in the work place is still marginal and if a woman wants to get ahead she's hardly likely to disappear once a month. I think the same would be true in most countries if women had such an opportunity.

Endometriosis has been labeled the career woman's disease because it was traditionally associated with working childless women in their 30s and 40s — endometriosis can contribute to infertility; however, many younger women, and those with children, also suffer from it. Having a child, as is sometimes recommended, does not necessarily cure endometriosis. The sexist connotation of this is that when a woman goes against her so called natural function of child rearing she'll get sick, any ambition to create in other ways being regarded as unnatural. Out with that idea!

Endometriosis, PMS and other menstrual difficulties worsen if you're stressed. The extreme sensitivity of your body could be alerting you to the unsustainability of current work practices, with all its stresses in today's economically rationalised, uncertain and environmentally polluted times. You just happen to have an immune system that won't put up with crap! If as a society we refuse to look deeply into things, our bodies will do the speaking for all of us.

Like the piece of grit in the oyster shell that creates the pearl, your symptoms are the irritant that can create the pearl of a more responsive and healthy workplace, and world for that matter. It's rather a tall order, but can you hang in with me on this idea? You were probably just wanting a quiet, unobtrusive life and now you've suddenly been singled out to be a general activist and troubleshooter!

You're probably thinking, "How the hell can my period pain make the slightest bit of difference, and if I were to get vocal about the failings of my work environment I'd probably be shown the door. I'm already seen as unreliable because I take time off for the pain, or I'm a no go zone premenstrually."

True, all true — I can't argue with you. But try this on anyway ... before the Berlin Wall came down no one imagined in their wildest dreams how it could be possible, and yet some dreamed of it, yearned for it, felt compelled in their own small ways to struggle for it.

Not being a historian I can't give you an explanation for all the historical forces in action at the time. But as someone interested in the power of the imagination and the resourcefulness of the human spirit to call up what seem like impossible alternatives, I do believe that apparently intractable situations can change. And it all begins with your wild, seditious, potent thoughts ... these are both seed and fertiliser for change. The Tao Te Ching tells us that "In the universe great acts are made up of small deeds". So play with possibilities — make tiny, tiny changes in the ways I've been suggesting. You won't look any different on the outside but you'll set in motion an internal revolution which, with the important ingredient of time, will also affect the external environment.

Your disturbances and symptoms are a call to sanity, to a more balanced way of operating. That's something to take a stand for. But to get well you don't need to broadcast either your suffering or your opinions on menstruation. And unless you work in a very supportive environment, I strongly recommend you don't! But you do need to make changes and attend to your physical environment. In some countries, such as Australia, occupational health and safety legislation provides some protection to employees. But you also have an obligation to take responsibility for your own health and wellbeing. I recommend you approach changes you want to make from a wellness viewpoint — as practising preventative medicine; because you like yourself too much to want to work in ways that are destructive to your body and soul; and because you want to stay well and work in physical environments that are healthy.

Are you happy, do you feel some meaning or purpose in your work that can sustain you? Is it a supportive place? Do you feel you have some control over and confidence in what you do? No amount of herb taking and vitamins will solve these dilemmas. Either you must leave work that is unsustainable for your soul, or find a way to achieve this. It's worth getting support with this one — talk to a career counsellor, to friends with whom you can brainstorm ideas, join a union to help you negotiate for a more equitable work place. Or talk to a psychotherapist to help you be more assertive or guide you to find meaning in your work. Find out whether your organisation has an Employee Assistance Program that provides confidential counselling to employees free of charge. Although these are long term goals, having made a choice to change jobs or improve the situation you're in you could be shocked at how fast it can happen sometimes. Just to take action can be empowering.

In the short term, the most important thing to remember is: be prepared for menstruation. By being aware of your cycle and accommodating your tendencies you'll dramatically reduce your problems. This might mean working extra hard leading up to the bleeding, and then keeping your diary as empty as possible during menstruation, taking extra care over your diet and thinking "tenderness" or whatever else it is that you want. If you're lucky enough to have flexible working hours, try to organise days off close to the bleeding.

If you have menstrual problems that cause you to take days off work, you'll have more of a challenge. Many sufferers of endometriosis have to do this because the pain will not bow even to a painkiller. And you may not want to take painkillers each month, recognising in the long run that they can create their own problems. You'll need to negotiate sick leave or leave without pay with your employer. Some can be very understanding and supportive of your need to work around your cycle. For example, you may be able to put in extra time in lieu of your day off. Some workplaces are more flexible than others and flexibility is what you need. An employer who values you may be happy to provide flexibility, knowing what good work you usually do.

Learning to appreciate the powers of menstruation can enhance your working life, not necessarily detract from it. Although you may come across negativity in the workplace towards your menstrual health needs, it's critical that you continue to try and negotiate for a healthier work environment, which will benefit everyone — including your employer!

The truth speaker

Twice Amy has done it. Feeling her rising ire at the injustices of her work situation she has told two different employers in no uncertain terms what she found intolerable. Amy, whose story appears in Restoring Imagination, can't afford to stop work at the drop of a hat. Her income, as well as her partner's, is necessary. But her need for justice won out. Both times she confronted her employers, Amy was prepared to lose her job. Both times she had forgotten she was about to bleed. And both times the blood appeared the following day.

On the first occasion Amy repeatedly requested regular weekly hours - particularly necessary for a mother. Her employers verbally agreed, but the promised regularity never materialised. Then after Amy's angry outburst her employers finally acted on their promises. She stayed on for another year, finally leaving because her freelance work began to take off.

Later she began work at a photographic salon, part of a chain, as a makeup artist. Not her ideal work but a gap filler over the summer months when all her freelance work would go into abeyance. Her first assignment was a young pregnant woman. The photographer made sleazy remarks throughout the session to the pregnant woman, leaving Amy feeling very uneasy. Despite feeling sick all over, she hesitated to say anything, thinking "I don't want to walk in here and be a bitch straight off." She suppressed her feelings until the day before her period when she realised "This is my chance to get my politics out there. I thought I always had to be on the fringe and run away." Her need to stand up for what she believed in outweighed all other concerns. She simply could not stop herself.

Being new to the company, Amy had no idea how they would react – to her surprise she had immediate and positive support. They showed concern about her complaints and insisted they wanted to employ people like Amy who cared about moral issues. As a result of this management alerted other salons to the incident and the unacceptability of the situation. Amy was also given the opportunity to state the conditions she needed in order to continue working there. A fairy tale ending perhaps. Nevertheless, Amy found the realities of negotiating with an all male management uncomfortable and is yet to see how it will unfold in practice.

It is the amazing force that arises in many of us premenstrually that sometimes makes it impossible for us to remain silent. It gives us the courage to speak out about our convictions. A breaking of the silence that can bring positive change where least expected.

4. *Handling Relationships*

Relationships, particularly a love relationship where intimacy can be deepest, are one of the best places to truly learn about ourselves and the world. Menstruation presents a curly relationship opportunity to women. Because of menstruation's demands for solitude it can seem to go against the needs of relationships.

If both parties are not aware of their respective needs and the overall health of their relationship, both the relationship and the woman's menstrual wellbeing will be affected. However, with awareness the menstruating woman can experience the relationship as a place of real support and, for both partners, the opportunity to deepen their connection with each other. Menstrual disturbance in a relationship is not the woman's "fault", as is often implied.

If a man is unaware of menstruation's imperatives he may inadvertently work against them. For example, if he wants to go out or wants attention and his partner feels a need to retreat. Yet, a man who knows how to appreciate the menstrual cycle will have an opportunity for evolution himself. If he can become more in touch with the right brain qualities of menstruation, to transform and "change his skin" as a woman does, his life will be more complete (Shuttle and Redgrove, 1995 p.71).

Few men are educated in the rhythm of their own physiology. I encourage a male partner to chart his moods and energy levels in conjunction with his female partner's cycle days. If he resists taking part in her cyclical changes his whole atmosphere will be opposed to them and he could be contributing to her PMS and other cyclical disturbances (Shuttle and Redgrove, 1995).

Women often tell me that once they begin living on their own, their menstrual problems ease considerably. If you want to live alone, that's fine. But equally, your menstrual disturbance can be used as an opportunity to make a positive impact on the world rather than forcing yourself to fit into the existing one.

If you do live with someone, and you both attend to your inner life, to feelings and dreams, in relation to the pattern of the woman's cycle, menstrual tension eases. I have found in that moment just before the blood appears an exquisite space for deepening closeness. A woman who feels supported in her deep solitary states is able to offer greater levels of intimacy and tenderness in relationship. A man who can support a woman and enter his own times of solitude with increasing ease offers the same.

A lesbian relationship may not experience the same tensions as a heterosexual one in this area because both partners know something of what it is to cycle. But because many women, both straight and gay, feel some ill ease with their bodies, and with menstruation in particular, difficulties may still arise. If either partner has difficulty being vulnerable or with expressing feelings, troubles could arise. Women who live or work together can also bleed together. This can result in either competing tensions or a cooperative, relaxed and tender time. In lesbian, as with heterosexual, relationships tension is eased with awareness and self care.

Valuing solitude in a relationship

In the premenstruum Jackie, whose story first appears in Depression, Loss of Meaning and Self Loathing, loses all perspective on life. "Things get blown right out of proportion — everything is an extreme". She cries, gets angry and reactive as well as depressed.

Jackie's instinctive need to retreat at menstruation was increased when she began her relationship, which has proved enduring and loving. But along with love came fear. That she wasn't good enough or deserving enough of love. Her self loathing was amplified in bucket loads just before she bled. It was scary for her and "freaked her partner out" — partly because her partner felt so helpless to support Jackie. Although her partner had her own menstrual problem, pain, she had no understanding of Jackie's premenstrual nightmare.

Talking to both her partner as well as to me has eased the terror for Jackie. Her partner understands not to take it personally and to respect that Jackie must simply take time alone, cutting communication with everyone. If Jackie can do this without self criticism her premenstrual anguish becomes manageable. As her life takes on more colour and richness, her premenstrual retreats become more a choice than a painful necessity. In time she may risk staying in with her partner during that time as an opportunity for deepening their intimacy. Her vulnerability is a gift to both of them because it provides the opening through which they can each reach a place of greater tenderness.

Relationships require give and take. I'm not suggesting when you're menstruating that you ask for special consideration that you wouldn't give to others. It's just that your partner needs to be aware that you are the one who is likely to need the primary consideration at that time. Not taking this into account is a recipe for conflict. Both partners need to exercise a little thoughtfulness!

Women do still tend to carry an unfair share of the feeling life of relationships, not to mention the cleaning, cooking and washing — men in Australia are still only doing about 30 per cent of the unpaid housework (MacKay, 1999). For many women the feeling and mothering role forms a large part of our identity — and we do it so well! Yet our skill at feeling and caring doesn't necessarily extend to a capacity for receiving tender feelings from others, or for allowing ourselves to be taken care of. Men generally do "the letting themselves be taken care of" part rather better than we do. At menstruation a woman is merely being reminded to take a leaf out of the man's book and ask, even demand if need be, that others do things for her for a change!

Relationships can have an inner life of their own. When the relationship is disrupted it's as though this inner life is speaking to us. Being only human we usually try to find a way to blame the other person for the disruption. For example, accusing them of being too much of this or not enough of that. Sometimes we're able to go further, to look into ourselves and do our own inner work so that we can learn more about ourselves and understand how we are contributing to the difficulty.

Although this is vitally important, the relationship itself is disturbing you because it wants **both** of you to pay more attention to it. The relationship may use one of the partners as its channel of communication. One of you starts to get restless, demanding, super vulnerable, jealous, angry. Although only one partner may be having these reactions, they are telling you something about the needs of the relationship, as well as something about yourself and your own psychology.

While it's necessary to use any disturbance as an

opportunity for self examination, our tendency to psychologise ourselves, or our partner, prevents us from dealing with the conflict as an activity of the relationship. The relationship is simply demanding us to engage with each other. It's telling us to talk with, listen to, confront, challenge, have a good argument. For the relationship to survive, you need to attend to each other as co-creators of the difficulty and its resolution, not as isolated individuals.

Your menstrual disturbances are a barometer for what's happening in your partnership. The partner who does not suffer, whether male or female, does a big disservice if he or she regards the menstruating woman's suffering as simply all her issue.

In Acting for the World I described how a menstruating woman becomes like a lightening conductor picking up unexpressed feelings. In a relationship she might be experiencing things which neither she nor her partner are attending to. Both parties may be unconscious of, or avoiding, some difficulty. Yet as the woman moves into the liminal space of the premenstruum she is more vulnerable to picking up the charge of unexpressed feelings of both partners. Perhaps she experiences it as an incoherent turbulence of tears, or as reactivity. With patience, respect and care on the part of both partners, the meaning of her distress will become clear and reveal invaluable information about the relationship.

I met one woman who was ready to divorce her husband at every period. Because neither she nor her husband were paying enough attention to the relationship, her feelings became more and more bottled up. Getting out of the relationship seemed the only solution when, in fact, more effective and honest communication may have been all that was needed.

I also remember a conflict brewing between myself and my partner. I was but a day or so from bleeding and I could hear a voice in my head saying "No. No. Don't say that, don't ..." But out the words came anyway — something very critical and the conflict escalated into a big fight. Unpleasant though the fight was, it heralded a breakthrough in our relationship. In my "ovulatory" world thinking, my "normal" mind, I would never have said out loud something so provocative. But I would think it nonetheless. Those thoughts can "white ant" away at a relationship and cause more hurt in the long term than a good healthy argument in the short term. Thank goddess for menstruation's provocativeness, challenging me to step out of my nice-girl-conciliatory-ways and making me more honest.

Remember that your partner, whether male or female, is not a mind reader, even though it may appear at times that they are. Always assume that they don't know what you're thinking or feeling. You need to say out loud what you're feeling or needing. Failure to take responsibility for your own feelings and needs results in confused messages which in turn can create conflict. Often women feel, particularly in the premenstruum, that her needs are not valid or important enough. Or worse still that there's something wrong with her for having particular needs. For example, that simple desire to be left alone, which may manifest itself as reactivity to everyone to get out of her path.

You need to take your own feelings, and those of your premenstrual or menstrual partner, seriously. Believe there's truth in what's being said even if it's discomforting to hear. You don't have to put up with what you feel are hurtful or unfair remarks but you need to deal with these in a direct way rather than simply telling her she's "just premenstrual". Saying this trivialises a real and meaningful experience. Say it in a dismissive way and you'll have an excellent strategy for escalating conflict on your hands!

As a partner to a woman with menstrual difficulties, be

careful that you don't focus on her as "the problem" and fall into "let's fix it" mode. You're not dealing with a malfunctioning machine — a human being likes to be understood not "fixed". Avoid using overly rational or logical arguments. As the partner you also need to be aware of how you could be focussing on her "problem" as a way to avoid the difficult feelings arising in you — you could be turning her into the problem to alleviate your own anxieties. In the end this doesn't work as failure to deal with your own reactions will directly aggravate the situation.

If you're receiving confused messages, ask your partner what she wants or needs. If she wants to be left alone, don't take it personally. Although it can feel like rejection sometimes, particularly if you're wanting or needing some attention from her, wanting time to herself doesn't mean she's rejecting you. Let her take her own time.

Menstruation itself may not always be the time to deal with relationship issues. For some women, the rawness or need for solitariness may be just too great to focus on the relationship. On the other hand, the power you feel at menstruation may make it the perfect time. But I suggest you don't make any dramatic decisions until your period has passed. You and your partner need to follow your own hunches, but don't continually avoid the disturbances once the smoother times of the month come round.

The strength of our sexual desire can wax and wane throughout the cycle and can become a source of tension if this is not appreciated. Ovulation can be a high point, but for some women menstruation can also be that. The sexual desire may be of a different nature at that time, perhaps wilder, hungrier, more sexually assertive. And yet for some women the idea of any contact feels strange, the need for genuine solitude overriding everything else. What is right is what imperative arises in you. Honour your own tendencies rather than performing for the other person.

Menstrual difficulties can disrupt your sex life — for example, women with endometriosis sometimes find sexual intercourse just too painful at any time of the cycle. Endometriosis sufferers also often have poor overall health which hangs about like an unwelcome third party in the relationship, demanding constant attention. This can truly wear down any partnership, and I have no easy answers. Your partner needs to be willing to embrace the perspectives I'm offering here, and to enter the difficulty less as "your problem" and more as opportunity for both of you to deepen connection.

This is asking a lot and some of you as partners might not feel up to it — or the relationship might not have enough going for it in the first place. If you find it too difficult to embrace the suffering of your lover, girlfriend or wife, be honest and talk about how it is for you. Don't judge yourself for not being able to handle it. I'm not sure I would have wanted to live with me through my nightmare years! Sometimes I think my partner had more acceptance than I did and I think the most wearing thing for him was my own subtle unconscious war with my body. Although I don't judge myself for that.

Clarity out of confusion

Katerina suffered from chronic fatigue and extreme, unpredictable bouts of pain from endometriosis. Working and living at home alone had its advantages in coping with her illness. But she wanted a long term relationship and knew her chances of conceiving a child were rapidly diminishing. At times she felt too sick to go out and meet people, and when she did, would have to take the whole of the next day off work to recover. She never knew if she would be well enough to attend social functions, making it difficult to plan anything. Because life was completely unpredictable, friendships, particularly new ones, were difficult to manage.

Because her illness often prevented her from taking part in social activities that would help lift her depression she became more and more isolated. She also didn't earn enough money to treat herself as often as she needed and her chronic fatigue prevented her from taking on more work to earn more income. A real catch 22!

Despite the seeming hopelessness of her situation she began in small ways to put changes in place that were healing (you can read about Katerina's healing journey in Nourishing Your Body). As she got stronger she met a man she was extremely attracted to and tentatively began a relationship with him. Should she tell him about her health problems? When would she tell him? Would he lose interest in her when he knew about them? Would sex be painful because of her endometriosis?

Of course all her health problems had to come out — they became apparent because she couldn't join in freely with some things, such as sharing a bottle of wine. At first the man was understanding, although she began to sense his increasing undercurrent of impatience because of the limitations in her life. As she put it "He didn't stop to think how hard it was for me missing out on some things, he was only aware of how it limited his life".

The relationship did not last and his final comment was that he "didn't want to go out with a woman who was sick all the time". Disheartening though it was for Katerina, he was at least honest and his reaction quickly revealed that he was not the man for her. Although it is understandable that a man would find it difficult to accommodate his partner's health problems, this particular man's intolerance for Katerina's poor health did not bode well for deepening intimacy and companionship, sickness or no sickness.

Although the endometriosis is still present to some degree, and possibly contributes to her recently discovered infertility, Katerina's experience of illness has fired her with more determination, clarity and ability to assert her own needs. She is working full time again and has an active social life including positive experiences of relationships. Both physically and emotionally Katerina is stronger — paradoxically it was the stress of this unsuccessful relationship that helped her find what she really wanted. She is now looking forward to adopting a baby from overseas and creating a family life as a single parent.

On the surface, illness has little to recommend it. It looks mainly like a serious impediment to all the things that apparently do hold value, like achieving in the world or your career. Yet trying to fight against, or deny, the suffering can turn up as tension and conflict in the relationship. Women who really face their illness, who take responsibility for their healing and who clearly assert their needs, usually find their partner is on side.

A better life

Penny, whose story I recounted in Initiation has severe health problems of which her endometrisosis is one feature. Her husband Greg, with whom she has been together for four years, is very supportive of everything she needs to do to build her wellbeing. When I asked him if he sometimes felt rebellious against the apparent limitations imposed by Penny's poor health, his response was a strong "No, I love her so much". He is willing to enter her world, and he takes care of himself by also doing lots of things by himself outside the relationship.

Rather than feeling hampered by the endometriosis it has opened opportunities to him. While already valuing his own health very highly, he's always open to learning new health practices. He realises that what's good for Penny is also good for him and his attention to his own self care motivates her to take care of herself. Attending support groups with Penny, Greg has found it useful to acquire knowledge about the illness — he has made it his business to understand all there is to know on the topic — and has listened to the stories of other women with painful symptoms.

Living in Sydney, both Penny and Greg had demanding jobs. Greg had his own awakening following a motorbike accident that incapacitated him for three months. When Penny's endometriosis was diagnosed, and she allowed herself to recognise how poor her health was, they both saw it as another catalyst for changing their lives. Greg got a higher paid job in another State and they found they could live a slower life in a cleaner environment with more opportunities for leisure and relaxation.

Penny loves the fact that Greg is so thoughtful, tender and caring with her. "He's a good doctoring person. But I don't want him to be my brother ... to be always in that caring mode thinking about me." She both wants and doesn't want that attention from him. She needs a balance in the relationship, to have a variety of roles, not to always be cast as the "sick one" and him the caring one.

The experience of endometriosis hit hard at Penny's sense of self worth. She doesn't like being ill and she doesn't like ill people. "Sometimes, on bad days, I feel I'm a big red wound, all diseased ... if I don't feel good about myself how can others? And I'm very thingy about the scars from the surgery" She has five incisions on her stomach and finds it difficult to be naked in front of anyone and is amazed that Greg would want to look at her scars at all. Although he can feel her rejection of her own body, he doesn't reject it and they have a good sex life. Although there is some pain for Penny with penetration, Greg is mindful of it and it doesn't affect their overall experience of sexual intimacy.

The emotional part is more difficult for Penny to cope with than all the physical "stuff". It has taught her to be more open about herself — in the past she would have put herself second in her relationships, now she "puts herself evenly". Although her menstrual symptoms have eased enormously, her suffering brought Penny and Greg closer together. This allowed them individually to examine their lives and to choose their future rather than drift aimlessly.

Ever the activist, Penny has gone on to form an endometriosis support group that empowers other women. She also challenges the lack of public health facilities in the area. Having made enormous advances in her healing Penny no longer has trouble with the colour red — she wears red cloth pads (the tampons are out!), red jewelry and red shoes.

Any kind of challenging experience, not just illness, will reveal the fault lines of a relationship. Like steel tempered in the fire you could both come out stronger. But without awareness, you may end up feeling just plain battered rather than tempered!

Menstruation is not an insatiable monster that everyone must bow to. Although if you don't attend to it, it can develop monstrous proportions! In relationships you can regard menstruation, which takes up a considerable chunk of a woman's life, either as a constriction or as a useful reference point for the vitality and resilience of your relationships. And an entry point to deepening intimacy.

Celebrating
the Genie

Women are blessed.

The menstrual cycle is our means to generate and regenerate. It allows women the possibility to create life. And all women, regardless of whether they suffer infertility, have the opportunity each month to renew their own body and spirit. Our cycle provides a means of inner referencing. And menstruation itself, an opportunity to come home to ourselves.

Our menstrual cycles are a great natural medicine!

The movements of the cycle are like the breath catching, like the snagging of threads in a garment. A sudden shift in gear, a cloud scudding across the sun, a small irritation, a distraction. Quiet, subtle, demanding our attention. Tripping us into different realities, perspectives and understandings. Breaking the mould of the cultural mindset. Stopping us from becoming rigid automatons and endless doing machines. Reminding us of ourselves and making us sensitive to the world.

It's the crucible in which we can forge internal authority. Attention to and acceptance of the conditions of the cycle cultivate that authority. Constant resistance or denial of the life of the body will lock us into an in-between-world: a perpetual adolescence of the spirit, an unripened emotional life.

The more rigid, linear and out of touch with the Feminine, with soul life and natural rhythms a culture becomes, the more severe will be the disturbance a woman experiences within her cycle. The menstrual cycle is both a monitor for her own wellbeing, and the world's.

If we know how to let go into the high sensitivity of the menstrual world, we have an amazing opening to greater intimacy and emotional maturity, to wisdom and altered states, to vision and ecstasy.

This is our power. A rich power, woven out of the strands of a woman's deep engagement with both inner and outer worlds. It emanates from our willingness to hold ourselves in dark and challenging moments. A mix of heart and head, instinct, intuition and intellect.

Most of all this power comes from our capacity to surrender. In that moment we can truly touch the awesome power of the Feminine.

Down to Earth

1. *Thoughts for a Power Woman's Travel Bag*

As you embark on your journey with the wild genie, remember to practise the following, according to your temperament and need:

★ Become interested in the whole of your cycle — chart it so that you know where you are at any given moment. Even if your cycle is irregular, chart the cycle you're having and see where it leads.

★ Write in your diary when your period is due and do only that which is essential. Think minimalism.

★ Know your tendencies around menstruation. Prepare for and support them.

★ Shop ahead of time so you have plenty of food in the house.

★ If your period falls on work days consider giving yourself a menstrual day off on your day off closest to the bleeding.

★ Consider keeping a dream diary. Notice if your dreams follow a cyclical pattern.

★ Ask yourself these questions: "If I could follow my natural inclinations leading into and during menstruation, without fear of judgment from others, what would I do? What is it I most want and need at that time?" Your reward for doing this will be freedom from suffering — great preventive medicine!

★ Be a little more unreasonable throughout your cycle rather than relying on menstruation to restore this useful quality to your life!

★ Please yourself more often.

★ Question whether you're taking on too much and therefore preventing others from doing their fair share. You may be blaming them unnecessarily for not taking on more responsibility.

★ Work out how others can support you. Remember that asking for support is the sign of an eminently sensible person.

★ Recognise that at menstruation you're meeting an aspect of your power. Meditate on the fact that you're a powerful woman and perhaps don't yet know how to use this power in the most effective way.

★ Try to respond more assertively to all those petty put down remarks about women, rather than pretend they don't matter. Even if you can't think of a quick reply come back to them wherever possible, minutes or even a day later.

★ Be prepared for any discomfort from others at your new found muscle flexing.

★ Find ways to exercise the sassy, punchy, mean parts of yourself in less threatening ways, such as play, role play or psychodrama. Find pleasure in any outrageous dreams.

★ Get to know your inner critic — listen for the particulars of how you put yourself down so that you can deal with your self-criticism better.

★ Don't forget, or ignore, what happens at menstruation only to be flattened by it again next time around. There is something about your symptoms that's giving a message about your life.

★ Do less. You don't have to give up on your life goals and dreams but recognise you're human, not superhuman. Allow yourself more time to reach those goals.

★ Ask yourself whether your goals are fuelled by cultural or family expectations. See your menstrual reactivity as helping you to go for what's important for you rather than what other people want.

★ Around menstruation, rest. Go to bed early, sleep in late and take afternoon naps. Fit in some extra dreaming time.

★ Find a simple ritual to mark the menstrual phase of the cycle.

★ Indulge yourself.

★ Practise tenderness, sweet tenderness. Cradle the raw, soft, putty-like you.

★ Avoid socialising during menstruation if it involves rich meals and lots of alcohol. You might want to avoid socialising altogether. People don't need to know why you're unavailable although you might feel comfortable to say that you simply want time to yourself.

★ Move at the pace of your body, rather than your mind.

★ Keep yourself warm when you bleed. If you suffer from cramping, avoid swimming in cold water although swimming any other time of the month is excellent. Avoid swimming in chlorinated pools.

★ Practise a little body awareness throughout the day. Notice where you're holding tension and work your body to release it. Let your belly relax and hang out.

★ Ease yourself slowly into an exercise plan. Walk more often as part of your daily routine.

★ Take five or ten minutes at the end of each day to just hang out with your body without distractions. Lie flat and simply notice the condition of your body and your breathing. Practise a simple relaxation routine.

★ Consider counselling or psychotherapy. Seek out a support group or form one yourself. It's great to have fellow travellers on your healing journey.

★ Draw on the power of menstruation. When you're bleeding feel your deep authority and work from that place.

2.   *Delicious Healing Recipes*

Home made remedies using everyday food items are a wonderful non toxic and inexpensive way to support overall wellbeing and ease menstrual problems. Make them a part of your daily routine.

Nettle Brew

Surprisingly tasty, this mineral rich drink is a great tonic.

Benefits

◄ excellent for strengthening kidneys and adrenals

◄ pick-me-up if you're fatigued

◄ stabilises blood sugar levels

◄ promotes healthy bones

◄ helps ease cramping and profuse menstrual flow.

The American herbalist and author Susan Weed speaks of nettle as a wonderful ally for women. She claims that two cups of nettle infusion daily will nourish and stabilise energy in the reproductive/hormonal systems, build nutrient rich blood and expand the cells' capacity to metabolise nutrients (Weed, 1989).

You will need:

A couple of handfuls of dried organic, or fresh, nettle

1 litre of boiling filtered water

Place the nettle into a lidded container. Add the boiling water and allow to steep for four hours. Drink the brew over one or two days and refrigerate unused portion. Nettle brew is a delicious drunk hot or cold — but don't drink it ice cold. If you don't have time to brew the nettle, make it the same way as you would a herb tea — just steep the leaves in boiling water for a few minutes.

Ginger Tea

Benefits

◄ aids digestion

◄ eases menstrual cramping and nausea

◄ helpful if your periods have stopped temporarily

◄ pick-me-up during the premenstrual tired phase.

You will need:

A small quantity of fresh ginger

Enough filtered or bottled water for one cup of tea

Finely grate the ginger (about a teaspoon). Add hot water and allow to steep for a few minutes. Alternatively cut some slices of ginger and simmer covered for 5 minutes.

Miso Soup (for one)

Miso soup, like the ubiquitous chicken soup is a panacea for all ills! Miso can be added to any soup or stew as seasoning, or you can try the following simple recipe. Include plenty of seaweed and you have an even more nourishing brew.

Benefits
- strengthening and alkalising properties

- helps the body resist disease

- full of lactobacillus (the same in yogurt) to aid digestion and assimilation of vitamins and minerals (as long as you don't boil it)

- promotes long life and good health

- treats and prevents radiation sickness

- neutralises some of the effects of smoking and air pollution.

You will need:
A handful of vegetables e.g. daikon (a long white radish), Chinese greens, pumpkin, carrots, green beans

1 inch strip of kombu, wakame or Tasmanian float leaf seaweed

Miso (brown rice miso or barley miso are good ones for soup)

A grating of ginger and/or shallots to garnish

One bowl of filtered or bottled water

Wash the seaweed and chop the vegies. Place the vegetables and seaweed in a pot with enough water for one bowl of soup. Bring to boil and simmer covered until the vegetables are just cooked. Remove the seaweed and cut it into thin strips. Return the strips to the pot. Put approximately half to three quarters of a teaspoon of miso into the bowl — experiment with the amount until you find the flavour you like. Add grated ginger and/or chopped shallots with a little of the hot liquid to form a paste. Then add the rest of the soup.

Miso in a hurry

Miso soup is a great way to start the day, especially in the premenstruum. If you're in a hurry, simply boil water and add to the miso for a miso drink. You can enhance this by adding a little grated ginger/chopped shallots/nori seaweed/crushed garlic. Delicious!

Caution: If you suffer from candida albicans (yeast overgrowth) and similar fungal infections use miso sparingly. Like other fermented foods, miso absorbs toxins from plastic containers, so store it in a glass, enamel or wood container (Pitchford,1993).

Soup stock

Yet another mineral brew — especially for those of you who are having trouble getting excited about seaweeds and enjoy eating a little meat and fish.

Make stock from the bones of meat or fish by covering the bones with water, bringing to the boil and then simmering on a low heat for approximately 20 minutes. Towards the end of simmering time add a teaspoon of cider vinegar. The acidity of the vinegar will draw the minerals from the bones.

Lemon Water

Lemon water is one of those all purpose remedies, which everyone can enjoy — always keep some prepared.

Benefits
◄   supports the liver

◄   aids digestion.

You will need:
One organic lemon

Two cups of filtered or bottled water

Roughly chop the lemon and place in a lidded glass container, such as a glass jar (the container must be glass). Add two cups of filtered or bottled water and allow to stand for two hours in the refrigerator before drinking.

Drink approximately a third of a cup after each meal and enjoy it at other times of the day too — especially if you're on a detoxification program. Drink a glass when you get up and your liver will be singing for the rest of the day! Also drink if you've been in polluted environments or feel a flu or cold coming on.

Rejuvelac

Rejuvelac is a fermented drink made from wheat sprouts. You can drink it straight or use it to make seed and nut cheeses and other ferments.

Benefits
◄ cleans the system

◄ improves the condition of the intestinal flora

◄ aids digestion and assimilation of vitamins and mineral.

You will need:
One cup of wheat grains

Nine cups of bottled or filtered water

First soaking: to one cup of wheat grains add three cups of bottled or filtered water and allow to stand for 48 hours (in hot weather this time can be reduced to 36 hours). Pour off the liquid.

Second, third and fourth soaking: use the same wheat grains. Add two cups of bottled or filtered water and soak for 24 hours. Pour off liquid after each soaking.

Rejuvelac should taste quite sweet, not sour. If it tastes unpleasant it's probably over-fermented.

One cup of wheat grains will yield approximately 9 cups of rejuvelac. Refrigerate rejuvelac that you don't use immediately. It will keep in the refrigerator for up to five days. After soakings you can eat the wheat grains, put them into bread or sow them to grow wheat grass.

Source: Kenton, S. and L. (9184) Raw Energy, London: Vermilion.

3. Luxurious Epsom Salt Bath

A hot bath with the lights low and a little gentle music is a time honoured way to get some psychic space, indulgence and quiet. Add some Epsom salts and you have got yourself an even more powerful remedy — while you're luxuriating in the hot water, your body is absorbing the magnesium from the salts. Magnesium is an essential mineral for all menstrual problems — including PMS, cramping, endometriosis, fibroids. It also helps to oxygenate the body and release toxins.

Take Epsom salt baths throughout the month, but particularly if you are very stressed, have been in polluted environments or subjected to heavy doses of electro magnetic radiation (EMR). Many of us work in air conditioned buildings filled with high-tech equipment and fluorescent lighting — conditions that can be wearing on the body. Along with fresh air, sunlight and exercise, Epsom salt baths are an excellent antidote. They're a boost for your immune system and so are also worth having if you feel a cold or the flu coming on.

There's an old wives tale that says it's not good to have a bath at menstruation. While these tales may seem nonsensical to our modern minds, there is sometimes a kernel of truth in these tales. Chinese medicine states that at menstruation a woman loses chi (energy). So it makes sense at menstruation to do only those things that build energy. Hot baths can be draining, particularly to those who have weak constitutions. Trust your instincts on this one!

Caution: Because there are so many chemicals in our water today, I would not recommend taking extended baths unless you have at the very minimum a chlorine filter (to remove chlorine) on your bath tap.

Indulging in the bath

It's particularly beneficial to have regular Epsom salt baths, say two or three a week. If you don't usually have baths, you'll need to build up slowly. Start by taking a bath for five minutes, then ten minutes and so on. Then when you can comfortably sit in a bath for 20 minutes, start adding the Epsom salts.

1. Heat the bath to approximately 40 degrees Celsius. This is a comfortable heat, but enough to cause you to sweat a little.

2. Add 4 to 6 cups of Epsom salts plus a handful of bicarbonate of soda. (the latter is optional)

3. Immerse yourself in the tub for at least 20 minutes.

4. Don't shower afterwards.

5. Lie down on your bed or the floor.

6. Cover yourself with towels to maintain your body heat.

7. Lie still for 10 minutes. You will feel a pulsation at the base of your spine which will gradually subside. This is the cerebral spinal fluid being pumped to your brain.

8. Enjoy your new sense of relaxation and vitality!

4.   *Warming Packs*

Castor oil pack

This is one of those old fashioned remedies that can be used for many different ailments. Castor oil packs are recommended for all types of period problems, especially endometriosis, fibroids and cysts, irregular periods or no period at all. Castor oil is also soothing for the nervous system and therefore ideal if you're unusually stressed, suffer from insomnia or have a tendency to colds and flu. Consider it for all that premenstrual bloating and crabbiness.

Castor oil packs improve immune system functioning, according to research from the George Washington School of Medicine. Castor oil packs have also shown improvements in the body's ability to both eliminate and assimilate vitamins and minerals, improve the functioning of major organs, glands and systems, improve lymphatic circulation and also draw acids and infection out of the body (A.R.E. Clinic, Phoenix Arizona). An all round winner!

Caution: I recommend you **don't** use the packs while you're menstruating, particularly if you bleed heavily.

Making your castor oil pack

You will need:

¼ to ½ cup of castor oil — preferably cold pressed and pesticide free

A piece of cotton or wool flannelette, folded into four thicknesses and large enough to cover your abdomen

A bath towel to lie on

An extra towel, folded, to cover the castor oil pack

Hot water bottle or heating pad

Castor oil pack holder (see Resources)

1. Soak the cotton or flannelette with castor oil. The initial soaking will use up to ½ cup of oil, later soakings will use less as the cloth becomes saturated with the oil. Eventually you can either wash the cloth or throw it away.

2. Place the soaked pad over your abdomen.

3. Put the hot water bottle, or heating pad, in the holder.

4. Place the holder on top of the pad.

5. Strap the holder and pad around your body to hold everything in place.

6. Cover the pack with a folded towel to keep in the heat.

7. Lie still for 30 to 45 minutes — enjoy, bliss out, dream into the experience or, if you are like me, fall in and out of sleep!

8. When you've finished with the pack, store it in the refrigerator.

The packs do take commitment. Start gradually — once a week for about 20 minutes, until you're familiar with its effect on you. Build up to three days in a row and then have a day off. If you're unable to do three days in a row, aim for three times a week. Keep this up for at least three or four months then taper off to once a week. Listen to what your body is telling you and adjust use accordingly.

Linseed pack

A little less messy, and cheaper, than castor oil packs, linseed packs don't take long to do. I can't personally testify to their efficacy for menstrual problems although I have used them to heal other health difficulties, such as constipation.

Making your linseed pack

You will need:

Approximately ⅓ cup organic linseed

Warm filtered or bottled water

A piece of cotton material to cover your abdomen

A bath towel to lie on.

1. Grind the linseed using a mortar and pestle. It's important to grind the seeds by hand as some of the healing and nutrient power is lost through electrical grinding.

2. Add enough warm purified water to make a paste.

3. Lying down on the towel, spread the paste over your abdomen.

4. Cover your abdomen with the piece of cotton.

5. Lie still for 10 minutes.

Start gradually — once a week for about 20 minutes, until you are familiar with its effect on you. Build up to three days in a row and then have a day off. If you're unable to do three days in a row, aim for three times a week. Keep this up for at least three or four months then taper off to once a week. Listen to what your body is telling you and adjust use accordingly.

The good oil

One woman I knew had not had her period for some time — her rhythms had been upset through an eating disorder. But while she had returned to normal, healthy eating and was on a special program of herbs and other supplements, her period would not return. Success finally came after she gave herself one castor oil pack treatment.

Dot had a prolapse uterus and at the age of 19 had an operation for it. Now in her early 40s she has endometriosis and fibroids. She has pain everyday, and bled for two months after a laparoscopy. She has been on the Pill for contraceptive purposes, with a few breaks, since her late teens. She now also uses it to manage pain, but with limited success. She began using Chinese herbs and acupuncture 18 months ago and had some improvement. More recently she tried using daily castor oil packs which proved to be very beneficial after only two or three months. Nine months later she is almost pain free.

5.   The Deer Exercise

The deer is renowned for its longevity and sexual energy, two benefits you'll experience from sustained practice of this Taoist exercise. It's especially beneficial for those women who suffer from menstrual problems. Not only does this exercise build energy, it balances the endocrine system, reduces and, in some cases, eliminates period pain. It can smooth out the premenstrual emotional bumpiness improve skin quality, reduce blood flow and strengthen the pelvic floor, anal muscles and rectum. Additional benefits include increased awareness of your body and even greater intimacy with yourself.

A winner at only 7 to 10 minutes a day! But like many healing practices, you'll have more success with this exercise if you focus your attention on it and practise it regularly. The exercise involves a gentle massaging of the breasts in a circular motion for a specific number of times. This is followed by a meditation to reabsorb the energy that has been generated into the body and balance the endocrine system. To do the exercise can feel like a prayer to your body.

Lisa Bodley has written a comprehensive and straightforward description of the Deer Exercise in her book *Recreating Menstruation*. She explains how the exercise works, answers typical questions about the exercise and describes women's experiences of doing it. Although you can learn how to do the exercise from the book, I also encourage you grab any opportunity to learn from a teacher.

6.   Catching the Blood

The risks

Disposable pads and tampons have been an incredible liberation for women. They have made menstruation a much less disruptive event, especially tampons. But for a price — both environmentally and personally.

Disposable pads in particular use up large quantities of precious and declining forest resources. According to UK based Women's Environmental Network (WEN), one fully grown tree makes only 500 disposable nappies. The pulp industry does use plantation softwoods, trees specially grown for the industry. But the mono-culture of these plantations can create a further set of environmental problems. According to the disposable pad industry, recycled material is not used because it lacks the long fibre — and necessary absorbency — present in virgin pulp (Pope, 1995). Reusable cloth pads, on the other hand, have years of use. One use items are decidedly uncool in these environmentally challenged times.

While dioxin, a highly toxic agent, is no longer used in the production of menstrual pads and tampons in Australia, a large number of other chemicals are involved to remove impurities and an ensure an effective absorbent agent.

The use of plastics in pads makes their disposal problematic — the modern disposable pad is not disposable because it's energy intensive to produce and not biodegradable (Pope, 1995). The plastics and synthetic material may create their own set of health problems. The plastic lining also makes it difficult for your vagina to "breathe" and could therefore possibly create a breeding ground for infection.

Disposable pads can also be irritating to the skin. Before I used reusable pads I would wear disposables — by the end of each period my vaginal area would be raw and tender. This never reoccurred once I began using the reusable cloth pads. Some women have also commented to me that they bleed less when using cloth pads.

Tampons present their own set of difficulties. Tampons are unsterilised, highly absorbent objects which absorb vaginal fluids along with the blood. A normal healthy vagina is the cleanest space in the body (Angier, 1999). Using tampons may interfere with the vaginal pH and may be implicated in pelvic inflammatory disease (PID). Tampons can lacerate the walls of the vagina, making your immune system — which already has enough to do in our polluted and stressful world — work harder, particularly if you suffer menstrually. Bits of fibre may also come loose and work their way into the uterus, causing infection over years of repeated use. Tampons are definitely contraindicated for any woman suffering from endometriosis or from period pain. Toxic Shock Syndrome (TSS), which has received a great deal of publicity, is relatively rare, although has swift and extreme consequences, including death.

The energetic and physical function of the blood actually flowing out of the body is, I believe, important. Wearing a tampon interferes with this natural flow.

The healthy alternatives

The safest product to use is the reusable cotton pad, ideally made from organic cotton. You would be doing yourself and the planet an enormous service by using them. When I first read about the pads I remember feeling a faint curling up inside myself. A momentary revulsion? Now I'm a devoted user and have never looked back, saving myself a considerable fortune into the bargain.

But while the initial reaction to cloth pads is not always favourable, once a woman has worn them something changes. I've heard countless stories of women finding that the reusuable pads are actually a breeze to use. Perhaps even more importantly, over time their feelings about menstruation become more positive. The reusable pads help make menstruation a little more special. And for those women who have strong environmental and political leanings, there's the warm glow knowing that they're not having to prop up a multi national each month! Cloth pads are generally made by small companies and individual women, sold in local health food shops, women's health centres and environmental centres or markets.

Some reusable cloth pads come with wings that clip underneath your undies much like some modern disposables. Others are more basic in style. The secret to safe and comfortable wear for all styles is in your undies — use them with snug, full brief cotton/lyrca undies and you'll wonder why you ever wasted your money on disposables all this time. The soft cotton of these pads is also so much more comfortable and you'll never run out.

It only takes ten minutes of your time at the end of your cycle to wash them. Soak the pads in cold water first until you're ready to wash them. It's wise to change this water regularly in warm weather, and always feed this soaking water to your plants — it's full of nutrients!

If you're a fit, healthy woman without menstrual problems you may get away with wearing tampons. But why wear your body down unnecessarily? I still recommend you sometimes use alternatives to tampons. The only type of tampon I recommend is one made from organic cotton, usually available in good health food shops. If your flow is not too heavy, you can use a natural sea sponge (soaked in bottled water for 24 hours before use to remove contaminants). After use soak in a non toxic cleaning agent or vinegar. Rinse the sponge and lay out in the sun to dry.

Another alternative for tampon lovers is the Keeper, a small rubber cup inserted in the vagina to catch the blood. Incredibly environmentally friendly, the only difficulty when you're out and about, and wish to empty it, is the need for a toilet and hand basin in the same cubicle. However it's contraindicated in women at risk of cervical cancer, or whose overall health is poor. If you like the idea of the Keeper I would recommend you alternate using it with pads.

Some women, with very strong pelvic floor muscles, are able to hold onto their menstrual blood until they go to the toilet when they release it. Women in some parts of Asia have been reported to do this. Although you can develop your pelvic floor muscles, you may not be able to do away with pads but you may not need as many and will avoid the risk of flooding. A simple way to start building these muscles is to tense and release the pelvic floor at least 100 times a day. So instead of getting impatient every time you have to queue or wait for something do the exercises! The more you do them the more you'll also heighten sexual sensitivity.

Using a combination of reusable and disposable according to the pace of their life suits some women. Initially you may not feel confident to be out all day with a cloth pad but when pottering around at home, why not give them a go? You could surprise yourself.

Be free — with pads!

Mainly a tampon fan, Madeline only occasionally used pads, for example, at night time. Then one day she had a day off work which happened to occur on the first day of her cycle when she usually experienced pain. She had been reading some positive literature on menstruation and decided that since she had this time to herself she would surrender to the process and also not wear tampons. She had no pain. Deciding to experiment further, she went back to tampons again the next cycle and once again experienced pain. That was enough evidence for her, she has now stopped using tampons altogether and continues to have pain free periods.

Her flat mate who was even more of a tampon fan than Madeline, never having worn a pad, discovered that her menstrual pain also diminished when she stopped using tampons.

7.   *Protecting Your Breasts*

The risks

The size of our breasts waxes and wanes throughout the cycle. I can always tell when I've ovulated because I suddenly become more aware of the presence of my breasts. They feel perkier and slightly fuller. This full feeling will sometimes increase as menstruation approaches, and they'll occasionally become quite tender. For some women this tenderness can be almost excruciating. In Traditional Chinese Medicine sensitive breasts are linked to a liver condition. But how much premenstrual breast tension is also the result of badly fitting bras? And how many bras do you know of move and grow with you from day to day?

Wearing bras has also been implicated in cancer. Medical anthropologist team Sydney Ross Singer and Soma Grismaijer based their findings on interviews with 4,700 women from five US cities. Women who wear a bra for 12 hours or longer every day are 19 times more likely to develop breast cancer than those who wear one for less than 12 hours. And women who wear a bra virtually all the time, even while asleep, are 113 times more likely to develop cancer as women who wear theirs for less that 12 hours a day. The bra, the researchers believe, artificially restricts the lymphatic system from flushing accumulated wastes from the body, allowing toxins to gather in the breast tissue which forms a breeding ground for a number of health problems including breast cancer (McTaggart, 1996). Regarded as controversial, and dismissed by the medical establishment, these findings nevertheless make sense as a contributing factor to breast cancer.

Wearing any kind of clothing that leaves marks on your skin is problematic as it means circulation has been impaired. For example, constriction at waist level impairs liver function. Underwiring in bras may also present another hazard beyond constriction of the lymphatic system. The World Health Organisation warned in 1987 and 1993 that the metal elements in spectacle frames constituted a health risk, acting as antennae and focusing ElectroMagnetic Fields around your eyes (Thomas, 1998). It must also be true then that the metal element in bras will do the same thing to the breast. In 1999 two women were killed when struck by lightening in Hyde Park, London. Their underwired bras acted as conductors, according to the Coronor (*Sydney Morning Herald*, 29 October 1999).

The healthy alternative

A Sydney based company, Full Bloom, has produced the Bodywise bra. It's designed to accommodate the normal cyclical changes in a woman's breasts. Made without underwire, hooks and eyes or heavy elastic, I can personally testify to their comfort. If this bra doesn't attract you, avoid underwiring at least for everyday wear. Make sure you get your bra properly fitted — if you find it leaves red welts on your body throw the bra out. Avoid wearing underwire bras while working at VDU screens. And whatever you do, don't sleep in your bra!

A friend of mine buys underwire bras and simply removes the underwiring. She finds the bras work just as well.

8.   *Light Matters*

For a healthy hormonal system, we need natural light in the day and dark at night. If you work in an office all day under artificial light, chances are you'll not be getting enough natural light. And if you wear sunglasses when outside, light reception will be further restricted and depletes the eye of Vitamin A.

We all need to take "sunlight baths" throughout our lives to maintain overall health. If you're not also getting enough Vitamin D from sunlight you won't be able to absorb calcium. Because some PMS symptoms are associated with calcium deficiency, this procedure, combined with a healthy mineral rich diet, can be very effective. If you suffer from lower back tension, eat more calcium rich foods and make sure to have the "sunlight bath" every day.

If you suffer from constipation it could be connected with poor diet and in particular insufficient calcium, which is required to promote peristalsis. So while making sure you have a diet high in vegetables, fruits and whole grains (avoiding excessive consumption of wheat and soy products) make sure you also get plenty of natural light.

Bathing in sunlight

As a minimum, expose bare arms, neck and face ideally for thirty minutes, between 7.30 to 8.00 a.m. if you live in the Southern Hemisphere, or between 8.00 a.m. and 8.00 p.m. during daylight hours in the Northern Hemisphere. Even if on some days you can't get the full half hour, at least ten minutes within this time is better than nothing. If conditions are unpleasant, such as rainy or cloudy weather, and you don't want to go outside, sit by an open window and wrap a blanket round yourself from under your arms to your feet. And if it's exceptionally cold, expose your face only, but double the time. Don't expect changes straight away — you may need to do this for at least 10 days before you notice an improvement.

If you spend most of your working life inside, make sure to get extra hours of sunlight on your days off. However, avoid prolonged exposure to the sun at midday. Eat plenty of chlorophyll rich foods which act as a form of stored sunshine and perform like vitamin D in the body to regulate calcium. (Pitchford, 1993).

Finding Extra Help

1. *Caring for Your Self*

An important part of self care is knowing when and where you need extra help. There are many therapies beneficial for menstrual problems — you may find you need a combination of different remedies such as herbs and chiropractic work; or kinesiology, naturopathy and counselling. Many of these therapies are now available in Australian cities and large regional centres. If there's no practitioner in your town, you may be able to gain some benefit by talking over the telephone to a counselor, naturopath or homoeopath.

Therapies to choose from include:

Acupuncture	Chiropractic
Homoeopathy	Herbs: Chinese and Western
Naturopathy	Kinesiology
Flower essences	Osteopathy
Orthobionomy	Remedial massage
Reflexology	Shiatsu massage
Reiki	Spiritual healing
Counselling	Music therapy
Art therapy	Psychodrama
Dance therapy	Yoga
Tai Chi	Qi Gong
Feldenkrais	

Therapies and health organisations

Australia

To find a qualified practitioner in your area contact:

Association of Remedial Masseurs
1/20 Blaxland Road
Ryde
NSW 2112
ph: 02 9807 4769

Australian Acupuncture Association
PO Box 5142
West End
Qld 4810
ph: 07 3846 5866

Association of Massage Therapists (NSW)
PO Box 1248
Bondi Junction
NSW 1355
ph: 02 9300 9405

Australian Association of Reflexology
2 Stewart St
Matraville
NSW 2036
ph: 02 9311 2322

Australian Hypnotherapists Association
FREECALL 1800 067 557

Australian Institute of Homoeopathy
29 Bertram St
Chatswood
NSW 2067
ph: 02 9415 3928

Australian Natural Therapists Association
PO Box A964
Sydney
NSW 2000
ph: 02 9283 2234
country and interstate
1800 817 577

Australian Music Therapy Association
PO Box 79
Turramurra
NSW 2074
ph: 02 9449 5279
email: information@austmta.org.au

Australian Osteopathic Association
PO Box 6999
Turramurra
NSW 2074
ph: 02 9449 4799

Australian Society of Clinical Hypnotherapists
30 Denistone Rd
Eastwood
NSW 2122
ph: 02 9874 2776

Australasian Society of Oral Medicine and Toxicology (ASOMAT)
PO Box A860
Sydney South
NSW 2000
ph: 02 9867 1111
fax: 02 9283 2230
(for safe removal of dental amalgam)

Australian Traditional Medicine Society
PO Box 1027
Meadowbank
NSW 2114
ph: 02 9809 6800

Chiropractors Association of Australia
FREECALL 1800 803 665

Shiatsu Therapy Association of Australia
332 Carlisle St
Balaclava
Vic 3183
ph: 03 9530 0067

PO Box 47
Waverley
NSW 2024
ph: 02 9314 5248

New Zealand

Association of NZ Ortho-Bionomists Inc.
PO Box 31-060
Milford
Auckland

New Zealand Association of Therapeutic Massage Practitioners
PO Box 375
Hamilton
email: nzatmp@ihug.co.nz

New Zealand Charter of Health Practitioners Inc.
PO Box 36588
Northcote
Auckland
ph: 09 4436 255

Umbrella organisation for all natural therapies.

New Zealand Register of Acupuncturists Inc.
PO Box 9950
Wellington
ph: 08 0022 8786
email: nzra@acupuncture.org.nz.

South Pacific Association of Natural Therapists
28 Willow Avenue
Birkenhead
Auckland
ph/fax: 09 4809 089

United Kingdom

General Council of Naturopathy
Goswell House
2 Goswell Rd
Somerset BA16 OJG
ph: 01458 840072
website: www.naturopathy.org.uk

Society of Homoeopaths
4a Artizan Rd
Northampton NN1 4HN
ph: 01604621400
website: www.homeopathy-soh.org

British Chiropractic Association
Blagrave House
17 Blagrave St
Reading RG1 IQB
ph: 01189505950
website:
www.chiropractic-uk.co.uk

General Council of Osteopathy
Osteopathy House
176 Tower Bridge Rd
London SE1 3OU
ph: 020 7357 6655

USA

The American Association of Naturopathic Physicians
PO Box 20386
Seattle
WA 98112
ph: 206 298 0125

The American Holistic Medical Association
6728 Old McLean Village
Dr McLean,
VA 22101
ph: 703 556 9245

Women's Business

Australia

Alexandra Pope
PO Box 1018
Bondi Junction
NSW 1355
ph/fax: 02 9310 0591
email: aepope@ozemail.com.au

I offer counselling and
psychotherapy for individuals and
couples, as well as workshops and
one on one sessions on menstrual
health and menopause. Phone
consultations are also available.

Amrita Hobbs
PO Box 337
Kyogle
NSW 2474
ph: 0419 336 291
email: amritahobbs@bigpond.com
website:
www.skyfamily.com/rediscovering-
rites

Amrita runs workshops in Australia
and overseas to support girls and
women through key life passages.
Current programs include: Girls
Growing Up (mother and
daughter, and father and daughter
programs); Rites of Passage (for
teenagers); Reclaiming First Rites
(for women); and Wise Woman
healing, a certificated training
program.

Diversity Counts
Shushann Movsessian
ph: 02 9386 5642
email: shushann@ozemail.com.au

Shushann offers counselling and
puberty workshops for girls from
9–12 as well as parent and
mother/daughter programmes. She
works privately and through
schools and the Royal Hospital for
Women, Sydney.

Felicity Oswell
PO Box 206
Manly
NSW 1655
ph: 02 9983 9440
email: felwm@ihug.com.au

Felicity, creator of the Wombmoon
Calendar, regularly runs Mandala
Moon workshops in Australia and
Japan using art and dance. She also
leads and teaches the Mandala
Dance of the 21 Taras and develops
Wisdom Moon programs for
women focusing on cyclic and
menstrual awareness.

Jane Bennett
PO Box 786
Castlemaine
Vic 3450
ph: 03 5472 4922

Jane runs A Blessing Not a Curse
workshops for mothers of
daughters from 8 to 12 years old to
prepare them for menarche.

Dr Karin Cutter, PhD
PO Box 5355
Port Macquarie
NSW 2444
ph: 02 6583 2961

Karin is a biochemist, naturopath,
homoeopath, herbalist and
nutritionist. She provides
consultation by telephone and
letter if you do not live in the area
and are unable to see her in person.

**Natural Fertility
Management**
Natural Fertility Management
The Jocelyn Centre
1/46 Grosvenor Centre
Woollahra
NSW 2025
ph: 02 9369 2047
fax: 02 9369 5179
website: www.fertility.com.au

National Coordinator: Jane
Bennett

This centre offers private
consultations and a correspondence
service for contraception, conscious
conception and overcoming
fertility problems. They also
provide a range of medical and
holistic therapies for reproductive
and general health issues.

**The International College of
Spiritual Midwifery**
The Balcony Room
Level 1, 210 Lonsdale St
Melbourne
Vic 3000
ph/fax: 03 9654 3737

Offer a range of seminars,
workshops, and individual sessions
on ancient women's knowledge in a
modern context: fertility, conscious
conception, childbirth preparation,
spiritual midwifery, healing,
women's mysteries retreats,
adolescent programs and much
more.

**Wise Woman Business
Pty Ltd**
Kerry Hampton
Fertility Awareness and Menstrual
Cycle Education

Kerry offers individual or couple
tuition, women only groups,
distance education, and mother and
daughter evenings.

PO Box 250
Canterbury
Vic 3126
ph/fax: 03 9830 5280

Women's Wilderness Quests
Maggie McKenzie
PO Box 42
Clovelly West
NSW 2031
ph: 02 9664 1968

Maggie, a psychotherapist, holds vision quests in pristine wilderness, including a three day solo, with full support and community. Quests offer a deeper connection with nature, self and life direction. They are also used to mark life's transitions.

New Zealand

Luna Collective for Women's Wellness
PO Box 836
Nelson
ph/fax: 03 5458 505
email: lunacollective@ts.co.nz
website: www.luna.tasman.net

This collective is non-profit and promotes women's health, in particular menstrual health. It produces information sheets and has menstruation and fertility resources.

Natural Fertility Management
Jo Barnet
220c Kilmore St, Christchurch.
ph: 03 365 1906.
email: herbald@xtra.co.nz

The Health Alternatives for Women (THAW)
PO Box 884
Christchurch
ph: 3796970
fax: 3663470
email: thaw@ch.planet.gen.nz

A health information and resource centre offering a variety of health services.

United Kingdom

Cabby Laffy
ph: 020 7482 6371
email: cabbylaffy@yahoo.co.uk

Cabby offers one on one and
couple counselling sessions as well
as group sessions and workshops on
fertility and/or sexuality, providing
practical and emotional support.

Natural Fertility Management
Carla Halford
1 Grove Cottage
Longnor
Shropshire SY57PS
fax/ph: 01743718951
email: carla@zesty.com

Women and Health
4 Carol St
Camden Town
London NW1
ph: 020 7482 2786

Resources and women's centre
offering low cost complementary
therapies.

USA

Ash Tree Publishing and the Wise Woman Centre
Susun Weed
PO Box 64
Woodstock
NY 12498
ph: 914 246 8081

This centre provides classes, books,
phone consultations.

Dr Christiane Northrup
12 Portland St
Yarmouth
Maine 04096
ph: 800 804 0935
website: www.DrNorthrup.com

Christiane is a medical practitioner
who also produces a newsletter,
information tapes and women's
health videos.

Menstrual Health Foundation
Tamara Slayton
708 Gravenstein Hwy North
PMB #181
Sebastopol
California 95472
ph: 707 522 8662
fax: 707 823 2137
websites: www.cyclesinc.org
www.e-irmc.org

Tamara offers educational
programs on coming of age,
menstruation and fertility cycles,
menopause, teacher training,
curriculum development and
program design.

Mysteries of Life
Judith Barr
PO Box 218
North Salem
New York, 10560
ph/fax: 914 669 5822
email: judbarr@judithbarr.com
website: www.judithbarr.com

Judith works with individuals and
groups worldwide. She teaches on
the feminine and women's
mysteries, including workshops on
menstruation, menopause and
sexuality.

Natural Fertility Management
PO Box 2215
Chapel Hill
North Carolina 27515

National coordinator (USA):
Joyce Stahmann
email: stahmann@yahoo.com
website: www.fertility.com.au

Orthobionomy
Zoee Crowley
1023 Makamua Street
Wailuku
Hawaii, 96793
ph/fax: 808 2429168
email: zoee@maui.net
website: www.maui.net/-zoee

Zoee is an orthobionomy
practitioner who also trains
orthobionomists worldwide.

Catching the blood

Australia

The Original Moonphase Period Piece (cloth pads)
PO Box 1018
Bondi Junction
NSW 1355
ph/fax: 02 9310 0591
email: aepope@ozemail.com.au

Distributor for northern NSW and Queensland
Full Moon
PO Box 91
Bellingen NSW 2454
ph: 02 6655 2696

Rad Pads (cloth pads)
PO Box 786
Castlemaine
Vic 3450
ph: 03 5472 4922
fax: 03 5470 5766
email: enquiries@fertility.com.au

**Wise Woman Cloths
(organic cloth pads)**
PO Box 250
Canterbury
Vic 3126
ph/fax: 03 9830 5280

Wemoon (cloth pads)
PO Box 249
Byron Bay
NSW 2481
ph: 02 6684 6300

The Keeper
PO Box 610
Harbord, NSW 2096
email: keepercup@hotmail.com
website:
www.morning.com.au/go/keeper

Sea sponges are available from selected health food stores and pharmacies.

Organic tampons are available in many health food stores.

New Zealand

Moontime Aotearoa (cloth pads)
Luna Collective for Women's
Wellness
PO Box 836
Nelson
ph/fax: 03 5458505
email: lunacollective@ts.co.nz
website: www.luna.tasman.net

Also available in most health food
shops around New Zealand.

The Keeper
PO Box 47820
Ponsonby
Auckland

Sea Sponges
Maree Hassick
Waiora Mara
Pokororo, RD 1
Motueka
ph: 03 5268829

United Kingdom

Ecofemme UK (cloth pads)
Dominique Pahud
15 Holmesdale Rd
Bristol, BF3 4QL
ph: 01179049726
email: dompahud@hotmail.com

Feminine Alternatives
18 Tor View Avenue
Glastonbury
Somerset BA6 8AF
ph: 01458 834787

Menstrual pads, sponges, fertility
information.

USA

Cascade Healthcare Products, Inc.
Moonflower Natural Products
Catalogue (cloth pads)
141 Commercial St. NE
Salem
OR 97301
ph: 503 371 445
fax: 503 371 5395
orders: 1 800 443 9942
website: www.1CASCADE.com

Gladrags (cloth pads)
PO Box 12648
Portland,OR 97212
ph: 503 282 0436
1 800 799 GLAD
email: b@gladrags.com

Menstrual Health Foundation (cloth pads)
708 Gravenstein Hwy North
PMB #181
Sebastopol
California 95472
ph: 707 522 8662
fax: 707 823 2137
websites: www. cyclesinc.org
www.e-irmc.org

Japan

Nawa Prasad (cloth pads)
3-15-3, Nishi Ogi Minami
Suginami - Ku
Tokyo 167 - 0053
ph: 03 3332 1187
fax: 03 3331 3067

Also contact point for women's
workshops run by Felicity Oswell
(see under Australia)

Nanohana (cloth pads)
22-75 Sekitacho
Tanaka, Sakyo - Ku
Kyoto City 606 - 8203
ph: 075 711 8264
fax: 075 711 5584

Ways Ltd (cloth pads)
376-102 Tamarucho
2 chome Senbonhigashi-Iru
Nakadachiuri-dori
Kamigyo-ku
Kyoto 602-8288
ph: 075 417-3546
fax: 075 417-3545
website: www.ways.co.jp

Healing products

Australia

Full Bloom Pty Ltd
PO Box 393
Paddington
NSW 2021
ph: 02 9361 6052, 1800 068 870
email: bodywise@fullbloom.com.au
website: www.fullbloom.com.au

Comfortable and attractive bras
and **those** leopard skin undies —
underwear for women of all shapes
and sizes including pregnant and
nursing mothers.

Aironic Pty Ltd
PO Box 216
Lane Cove
NSW 2066
ph: 02 9439 7599

Ionisers for home and car (worth
getting especially if your health is
poor and/or you do a lot of
driving).

Pesticide free castor oil and pack holder
You may find these at selected
health practitioners or you can
import your own from The
Heritage Store, USA (see below).

USA

Avena Botanicals
219 Mill St
Rockport
Maine 04856
ph: 207 594 0694

Women owned and run, this
organisation provides organic herbs
and products, classes and cloth
pads.

Cascade Healthcare Products, Inc.
Moonflower Natural Products
Catalogue (herbs and products for
babies and women) and the Birth
and Life Bookstore Catalogue

141 Commercial St. NE
Salem
OR 97301
ph: 503 371 445
fax: 503 371 5395
orders: 1 800 443 9942
website: www.1CASCADE.com

Mountain Rose Herbs
20818 High St
North San Juan
CA 95960
ph: 800 879 3337
website: www.botanical.com/mtrose

This company will ship
internationally.

The Heritage Store
Dept C
PO Box 444
Virginia Beach
VA 23458-0444
ph: 757 428 4941
fax: 757 428 3632
email: heritage@caycecures.com

Supply pesticide free castor oil and
pack holder.

Support groups and organisations

Australia

DES (diethylstilboestrol) support
PO Box 282
Camberwell
Vic 3124
ph: 03 9870 0536

14 Edmundson Close
Thornleigh
NSW 2120
ph: 02 9875 4820

Endometriosis Complementary Therapies Support Group
Lorraine Henderson
ph: 0418 177 951

Endometriosis Support Group
Royal Hospital for Women
Barker St
Randwick
NSW 2031
ph: 02 9382 6700

Endometriosis Association NSW
Hemsley House
20 Roslyn St
Potts Point
NSW 2011
ph: 02 9356 0450
fax: 02 9357 2334

Endometriosis Association VIC
37 Andrew Cres
South Croydon
Vic 3136

Endometriosis Support Group QLD
Penny Fenton
ph: 07 5521 0507

Women's Community Health Centres —
check telephone directory or state government health department for a centre in your area

Women's Health Victoria
ph: (03) 9662 3755
Health Information Line:
03 9662 3742
email: whv@whv.org.au.
website: www.whv.org.au

New Zealand

DES (diethylstilboestrol) support
Prof. Charlotte Paul
Preventative and Social Medicine
Otago Medical School
Box 913
Dunedin

New Zealand Endometriosis Foundation
PO Box 1683
Palmerston North
ph/fax: 06 3592613
email: nzendo@xtra.co.nz.
website: www.nzendo.co.nz.

United Kingdom

DES (diethylstilboestrol) support
c/- NWCI
16-20 South Cumberland St
Dublin 2

DES (diethylstilboestrol) support
c/- Women's Health (see below)

Endometriosis Society Helpline
ph: 020 7222 2776

National Association for Premenstrual Syndrome
7 Swift's Ct
High St
Seal
Kent TN15 OEG

PO Box 72
Sevenoaks
Kent TN13 1XQ
ph/fax: 01732760011
helpline: 01732760012
email: naps@charity.vfree.com
website: www.pms.org.uk

The Menopause Helpline Ltd
228 Muswell Hill
Broadway
London N10 3SH
ph: 020 8444 5202
fax: 020 8444 6442

Offers support for women suffering from side effects of HRT and the Pill.

Women's Health
52 Featherstone St
London EC1Y 8RT
ph: 020 7251 6580
website:
www.womenshealthlondon.org.uk

A resource, information and support centre.

United States

DES (diethylstilboestrol) support
US National Office
610 - 16th St #301
Oakland
CA 94612
ph: 1 800 DES 9288 or
510 465 4011.
fax: 510 465 4815
email: desact@well.sf.ca.us

Canada

DES (diethylstilboestrol) support
National Office
5890 Monkland, Suite 203
Montreal
Quebec H4A 1G2

Websites

www.laraowen.com
www.menstruation.com
www.endometriosisassn.org

2. Caring for Your Environment

Environmentally friendly organisations

Australia

Chemfree Cleaning
C/- Cleanhouse Effect
445 King Street
Newtown
NSW 2042
mobile: 0403 179819

Cleanhouse Effect shops (Planet Ark)
445 King St
Newtown
NSW 2042
ph: 02 9516 4681

37 Cantonment Street
Fremantle
WA 6160
ph: 08 9430 5054
(also sell cloth pads)

Enviro-Tru
14 Mort Street
Katoomba NSW
ph: 02 4782 5375
website:
www.truebluegreen.com/envirotru
email: azura@pnc.com.au

Offers mail order service for environmentally friendly cleaning products.

Systems Pest Management
1/27a Oxford St
Epping
NSW
ph: 02 9865 5288.

This company provides alternative pest extermination and has strict standards. If you don't live in their area, speak to them for guidance or check the internet, your local environment center or health food shop. Standards vary widely between companies so be wary.

Total Environment Centre
Level 2, 362 Kent St
Sydney
NSW 2000
ph: 02 9299 5599
fax: 02 9299 4411.
website: www.tec.ncccnsw.org.au

Working Women's Centre
157 Wardell Street
Dulwich Hill, NSW
ph: 02 9559 5355

National Occupational Health and Safety Commission
92 Parramatta Rd
Camperdown
NSW
ph: 02 9577 9555
website: www.nohsc.gov.au

United Kingdom

Women's Environmental Network
PO Box 30626
London E1 1TZ
ph: 020 7481 9004
email: wenuk@gn.apc.org
website: www.gn.apc.org/wen

Organically grown produce

Australia

Mooneys
PO Box 352
Port Macquarie
NSW 2444
ph: 02 6583 7883
fax: 02 6583 2235

If you have difficulty finding
organic food locally, Mooneys
deliver biodynamic and organic
produce around Australia free with
a minimum order.

**The National Association for
Sustainable Agriculture,
Australia (NASAA)**
Head Office:
PO Box 768
Stirling
SA, 5152
ph: 08 370 8455
fax: 08 370 8381

This association will help you find
a supplier in your area.

**Australian Gen-ethics
Network**
c/o 340 Gore Hill
Fitzroy
Vic 3065
ph: 03 9416 2222

Provides information about genetic
engineering and genetically
modified food.

New Zealand

BIOGRO
PO Box 9693
Marion Square
Wellington
ph: 04 8019741
fax: 04 8019742
email: info@bio-gro.co.nz

Fairground Eco Store
PO Box 91718
AMSC
Auckland
ph/fax: 09 3768 577 or
08 0077 3247

Provide mail order service.

Soil and Health Association
PO Box 36170
Northcote
Auckland
ph/fax: 09 4804440
email: soil@health.pl.net

United Kingdom

The Soil Association
Bristol House
40-46 Victoria Street
Bristol, BS1 6BY
ph: 0117 9290661
website: www.soilassociation.org.uk

Provides a directory of organic
food suppliers in your area.

References

Revealing the Jewel

Crook, W.G. (1986) *The Yeast Connection: A Medical Breakthrough*, New York: Vintage Books.

Grahn, J. (1993) *Blood Bread and Roses, How Menstruation Created the World*, Boston: Beacon Press Books.

Greer, G. (1999) *The Whole Woman*, London: Doubleday.

Hillman, J. and Ventura, M. (1992) *We've Had 100 Years of Psychotherapy and the World's Getting Worse*, New York: Harper Collins

Leviton, R. "Rossi Rhythm: the Rhythms of Life", *Wellbeing Magazine*, No. 62, December 1995.

Siegel, B. (1988) *Love, Medicine and Miracles*. London: Arrow Books.

Walker, B. (1983) *The Woman's Encyclopedia of Myths and Secrets*, New York: Harper Collins.

Weill, A. (1995) *Spontaneous Healing*. New York: Ballantine Books.

Restoring Imagination

Shuttle, P. and Redgrove P. (1986) *The Wise Wound*. London: Paladin.

Initiation

Borysenko, J. (1996) *A Woman's Book of Life: The Biology, Psychology and Spirituality of the Feminine Life Cycle*. New York: Riverhead Books.

Buckley, T. and Gottlieb, A. (eds) (1988) *Blood Magic: the Anthropology of Menstruation*. Berkeley: University of California.

From *Blood Bread and Roses* by Judy Grahn, Copyright , 1993 by Judith Rae Grahn. Reprinted by permission of Beacon Press, Boston.

Owen, L. (1993) *Her Blood is Gold*. San Francisco: Harper Collins.

Sardello, R. (1995), *Love and the Soul: Creating a Future for Earth*, New York: Harper Collins

Saul J.R. (1997) *The Unconscious Civilisation*, Ringwood: Penguin.

Slayton, T. (1990) *Reclaiming the Menstrual Matrix: Evolving Feminine Wisdom*. Santa Rosa: Menstrual Health Foundation.

Tacey, D. (1997) *Remaking Men: The Revolution in Masculinity*. Ringwood: Penguin Australia.

Tacey, D. (1999) *Soul of Australia and the Republic Forum*. Sydney.

Walker, B. (1983) *The Woman's Encyclopedia of Myths and Secrets*, New York: Harper Collins.

Weill, A. (1995) *Spontaneous Healing*. New York: Ballantine Books.

Listening to Yourself

Angier, N. (1999) *Woman: An Intimate Geography*. London: Virago.

Borysenko, J. (1996) *A Woman's Book of Life: The Biology, Psychology and Spirituality of the Feminine Life Cycle*. New York: Riverhead Books.

DesMaisons, K. (1999) *Potatoes Not Prozac*. New York: Simon and Schuster

Hall, N. (1980) *The Moon and The Virgin*. New York: Harper & Row

Hartmann, E. (1967) *The Biology of Dreaming*. Boston: Charles C Thomas.

Pinkola Estes, C. (1992) *Women Who Run with the Wolves*, London: Rider.

Shuttle, P. and Redgrove P. (1986) *The Wise Wound*. London: Paladin

Sydney Morning Herald, The Good Weekend, 31 July 1999 (article title?)

Shuttle, P. and Redgrove P. (1995) *Alchemy for Women: Personal Transformation Through Dreams and the Female Cycle*. London: Rider.

Using the Power of Menstruation

Leyden-Rubenstein, L.A. (1998) *The Stress Management Handbook: Strategies for Health and Inner Peace*. New Canaan: Keats Publishing Inc.

Owen, L. "The Sabbath of Women" *Whole Earth Review*, Summer 1991.

Owen, L. (1993) *Her Blood is Gold*. San Francisco: Harper Collins.

Owen, L. (1998) H*onoring Menstruation: A Time of Self Renewal*. California: The Crossing Press.

Robbins T. (1980) *Still Life With Woodpecker*, Toronto: Bantam.

Weed, S. (1992) *Menopausal Years: the Wise Woman Way, Alternative Approaches for Women 30-90*. Woodstock: Ash Tree Publishing.

Nourishing Your Body

Naish, F. (1993) *Natural Fertility: the Complete Guide to Avoiding or Achieving Conception*. Burra Creek: Sally Milner Publishing.

Pitchford, P. (1993) *Healing with Whole Foods*, Berkeley: North Atlantic Books.

Weed, S. (1989) *Healing Wise*, Woodstock: Ash Tree Publishing.

Menstruation the World and You

Kenton, S. and L. (9184) *Raw Energy*, London:Vermilion.

McTaggart, L. *What Doctors Don't Tell You*, Vol. 7 No. 1, 1996.

Mooncircle Teaching — Minisa Crumbo Creek — Pootawatomi. Contact: Brush Dance, 218 Cleveland Court, Mill Valley, CA 94941.

Pitchford, P. (1993) *Healing with Whole Foods*, Berkeley: North Atlantic Books.

Pope, A. "The Hidden Hazards of Menstrual Hygiene" *Australian Wellbeing Magazine*, 1995 Annual (Collectors' Edition), No. 58.

Sydney Morning Herald, 29 October 1999.

Thomas, P. (1998) *What Doctors Don't Tell You*, Vol. 9, No. 6, 1998.

Down to Earth

Pitchford, P. (1993) *Healing with Whole Foods*, Berkeley: North Atlantic Books.

Pope, A. "The Hidden Hazards of Menstrual Hygiene" *Australian Wellbeing Magazine*, 1995 Annual (Collectors' Edition), No. 58.

Weed, S. (1989) *Healing Wise*, Woodstock: Ash Tree Publishing.

Further Reading

More on the amazing world of menstruation

Buckley, T. and Gottlieb, A., (eds.) (1988) *Blood Magic: The Anthropology of Menstruation.* Berkeley and Los Angeles: University of California.

Cameron, A. (1981) *Daughters of Copper Woman.* Vancouver: Press Gang.

Golub, S. (1992) *Periods: From Menarche to Menopause.* Newbury Park: Sage Publications.

Grahn, J. (1993) *Blood, Bread and Roses: How Menstruation Created the World.* Boston: Beacon Press.

Knight , C. (1991) *Blood Relations: Menstruation and the Origins of Culture.* New Haven: Yale University Press.

Owen, L. (1998) *Honouring Menstruation: A Time of Self Renewal.* Freedom: Crossing Press.

Shuttle, P. and Redgrove, P. (1989) *The Wise Wound.* London: Paladin

Shuttle, P., and Redgrove, P. (1995) *Alchemy for Women: Personal Transformation Through Dreams and the Female Cycle.* London: Rider.

Some really healthy books

Bays, B. (1999) *The Journey: Extraordinary Guide to Healing Life and Setting Yourself Free*. London: Thorsons.

Bodley, L.(1995) *Recreating Menstruation*. Melbourne: Gnana Foundation (only available from PO Box 246, Yarra Junction, Victoria 3797, Australia. Email: lisa@gnanayoga.com.au)

Brown, S. (1996) *Better Bones, Better Body*. New Canaan: Keats Publishing, Inc.

Epstein, S. and Steinman, D. (1997) *The Breast Cancer Prevention Program*. New York: Macmillan.

Gray, M. (1994) *Red Moon: Understanding and Using the Gifts of the Menstrual Cycle*. Brisbane: Element Books Ltd.

Krohn, J., Taylor, Frances A. and Prosser J. (1996) *The Whole Way to Natural Detoxification: The Complete Guide to Clearing Your Body of Toxins*. Point Roberts: Hartley and Marks Publishing Inc.

Lark, S.M. (1984) *PMS:Premenstrual Syndrome Self Help Book*. Berkeley: Celestial Arts.

Lark, S.M. (1993) *Menstrual Cramps: A Self Help Program*. Los Altos: Westchester Publishing Company.

Leyden-Rubenstein, L.A. (1998) *The Stress Management Handbook: Strategies for Health and Inner Peace*. New Canaan: Keats Publishing Inc.

McTaggart, L. (1996) *What Doctors Don't Tell You: The Truth About the Dangers of Modern Medicine*. London: Thorsons.

Naish, F. (1991) *Natural Fertility*. Burra Creek: Sally Milner Publishing.

Naish, F. and Roberts, J. (1996) *The Natural Way to Better Babies: Preconception Health Care for Prospective Parents*. Sydney: Random House.

Northrup, C. (1995) *Women's Bodies, Women's Wisdom*. London: Piatkus.

Pitchford, P. (1993) *Healing with Whole Foods*. Berkeley: North Atlantic Books.

Trickey, R. (1998) *Women, Hormones and The Menstrual Cycle: Herbal and Medical Solutions from Adolescence to Menopause*. St Leonards: Allen and Unwin.

Trickey, R. and Cooke, K. (1998) *Women's Trouble: Natural and Medical Solutions*. St Leonards: Allen and Unwin.

Weed, S. (1989) *Healing Wise*. Woodstock: Ash Tree Publishing.

Weed, S. (1992) *Menopausal Years: The Wise Woman Way, Alternative Approaches for Women 30-90*. Woodstock: Ash Tree Publishing, 1992

What Doctors Don't Tell You, Satellite House, 2 Salisbury Rd, London, SW19 4EZ. Email: wddty@zoo.co.uk. Website: www.wddty.co.uk (an informed, useful monthly health publication).

Healthy environments

Baggs, S. and Baggs, J. (1996) *The Healthy House: Creating a Safe, Healthy and Environmentally Friendly Home*, Sydney: HarperCollins Publishers.

Dadd, D.L. (1997) *Home Safe Home: Protecting Yourself and Your Family from Everyday Toxics and Harmful Household Products*. New York: Jeremy P Tarcher/Putnam.

Both the above books have excellent resource lists.

Exploring women's matters

Angier, N. (1999) *Woman: An Intimate Geography*. London: Virago.

Borysenko, J. (1996) *A Woman's Book of Life: the Biology, Psychology and Spirituality of the Feminine Life Cycle*. New York: Riverhead Books.

Ehrenreich, B. and English, D. *Witches, Midwives and Nurses: A History of Women Healers*. New York: The Feminist Press. (no year given)

George, D. (1992) *Mysteries of the Dark Moon: The Healing Power of the Dark Goddess*. San Francisco: Harper Collins.

Hall, N. (1980) *The Moon and The Virgin: Reflections on the Archetypal Feminine*. New York: Harper and Row.

Harding, M.E. (1990) *Women's Mysteries, Ancient and Modern*. Boston: Shambhala.

Kirner, J., and Rayner, M. (1999) *The Woman's Power Handbook*. Ringwood: Penguin.

Lawrence, L. and Weinhouse, B. (1997) *Outrageous Practices: How Gender Bias Threatens Women's Health*. New Brunswick: Rutgers University Press.

Martin, E. (1992) *The Woman in the Body: A Cultural Analysis of Reproduction*. Boston: Beacon Press.

Mookerjee, A. (1988) *Kali, The Feminine Force*. Rochester, VT: Destiny Books.

Noble, V. (1981) *Motherpeace: A Way to the Goddess through Myth, Art and Tarot*. San Francisco: Harper Collins.

Sjoo, M. and Mor, B. (1991) *The Great Cosmic Mother: Recovering the Religion of the Earth*. San Francisco: Harper Collins.

Walker, B. (1983) *The Woman's Encyclopaedia of Myths and Secrets*. San Francisco: Harper Collins.

Ussher, Jane M. *The Psychology of the Female Body*. London and New York: Routledge, 1989.

Food for soul, inner life and relationships

Hillman, J. (1996) *The Soul's Code: In Search of Character and Calling*. New York: Random House.

Mindell, A. (1993) *The Shaman's Body: a New Shamanism for transforming health, relationships and community*. New York: Harper Collins.

Mindell, A. (1985) *Working with the Dreaming Body*. London: Routledge and Kegan Paul.

Mindell, A. (1990) *Working on Yourself Alone*. London: Arkana.

Moore, T. (1992) *Care of the Soul.* New York: Harper Collins.

Sardello, R. (1995) *Love and the Soul: Creating a Future for Earth.* New York: Harper Collins.

Sardello, R.(1992) *Facing the World with Soul: the Reimagination of Modern Life.* Hudson: Lindisfarne Press.

Sardello, R. (1999) *Freeing the Soul from Fear.* New York: Riverhead Books.

Schnarch, D. (1997) *Passionate Marriage: Keeping Love and Intimacy Alive in Committed Relationships.* Melbourne: Scribe Publications.

Index